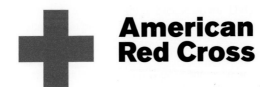

American Red Cross

Family Caregiving

StayWell®

A MediMedia USA Company

Dedication

This book and DVD are dedicated to the millions of family caregivers who respond with love and compassion when a loved one needs their help.

Note to Our Readers

This book and the accompanying DVD are not intended as a substitute for professional medical care, legal or financial advice. You should seek such advice from medical, legal and financial professionals.

This book and the accompanying DVD are not a substitute for materials used in American Red Cross courses in which First Aid or CPR certification is given.

Family caregivers care for both men and women. Rather than say "he or she" and "him or her" each time, we alternate the gender reference throughout the text.

When you see this DVD icon ⓞ in the book margins, it means the skill is demonstrated or the topic is covered in greater detail on the enclosed DVD.

Copyright © 2007 by The American National Red Cross

All rights reserved. No part of this publication may be reproduced, stored in a retrieval system or transmitted in any form or by any means, electronic, mechanical, photocopying, recording or otherwise, without prior permission from American Red Cross National Headquarters, Products and Health and Safety Services.

Design and production by Tutto Design and Communications, Newtown, PA
Printed in China
StayWell
780 Township Line Rd.
Yardley, PA 19067

ISBN-10 1-58480-391-6
ISBN-13 978-158480-391-1

Library of Congress Cataloging-in-Publication Data is available from the publisher.

06 07 08 09 10 9 8 7 6 5 4 3 2 1

About the American Red Cross

Mission of the American Red Cross
The American Red Cross, a humanitarian organization led by volunteers and guided by its Congressional Charter and the Fundamental Principles of the International Red Cross Movement, will provide relief to victims of disaster and help people prevent, prepare for, and respond to emergencies.

The American Red Cross has helped people mobilize to help their neighbors for 125 years. In 2005, victims of a record 72,883 disasters, most of them fires, turned to the nearly 1 million volunteers and 35,000 employees of the Red Cross for help and hope. Through more than 800 locally supported chapters, more than 15 million people each year gain the skills they need to prepare for and respond to emergencies in their homes, communities and world. Almost 4 million people give blood—the gift of life—through the Red Cross, making it the largest supplier of blood and blood products in the United States. The Red Cross helps thousands of U.S. service members, separated from their families by military duty, stay connected. As part of the International Red Cross and Red Crescent Movement, a global network of more than 180 national societies, the Red Cross helps restore hope and dignity to the world's most vulnerable people. An average of 91 cents of every dollar the Red Cross spends is invested in humanitarian services and programs. The Red Cross is not a government agency; it relies on donations of time, money and blood to do its work.

Fundamental Principles of the International Red Cross
and Red Crescent Movement
Humanity
Impartiality
Neutrality
Independence
Voluntary Service
Unity
Universality

Acknowledgments

This *Family Caregiving* book and DVD set was developed and produced through the combined efforts of the American Red Cross, external reviewers and StayWell. Without the commitment to excellence of both paid and volunteer staff, this product could not have been created.

The American Red Cross team for this product included: Scott Conner, Vice President, Products and Health and Safety Services; Don Vardell, National Chair, Products and Health and Safety Services; Pat Bonifer and Steve Rieve, Directors; Emilie Parker, Project Manager; Marc Madden and Adreania McMillian, Senior Associates; Jean Erdtmann, Officer, Sales Support and Business Capacity Development; Greta Petrilla, Communications and Marketing Manager; Betty Butler, Administrative Assistant; and Rhadames Avila, Administrative Associate.

The StayWell Team included: Nancy Monahan, Senior Vice President; Bill Winneberger, Senior Director of Manufacturing; Paula Batt, Executive Director, Sales and Business development; Reed Klanderud, Executive Director, Marketing and New Product Development; Beverly Payton, Developmental Editor; and Stephanie Weidel, Senior Production Editor.

The American Red Cross and StayWell thank: Alternatives NY, Advertising and Design Agency; Rick Brady, photographer; Dan Cartledge, copy editor; Brenna McDonough, actress; Karen M. Ruppert, proofreader; Glenn Shockley, LMA Digital; David Spagnolo, cover photographer; and Rosemary Tottoroto, graphic designer; for their contributions to the production of this book and DVD.

The following members of the American Red Cross Advisory Council on First Aid and Safety also provided guidance and review:

David Markenson, M.D., FAAP, EMT-P
Chair, American Red Cross Advisory Council on First Aid and Safety
Chief, Pediatric Emergency Medicine
Maria Fareri Children's Hospital
Westchester Medical Center
Valhalla, New York

Donald J. Gordon, Ph.D, M.D.
Member, American Red Cross Advisory Council on First Aid and Safety
Professor, DEMT, UTHSC-SA
EMS Medical Director
San Antonio, Texas

The following people and organizations provided expert review of the materials and support for *Family Caregiving*:

Mitchell Berdiey, Psy.D
Associate Director, Pro Behavioral Health Inc., Denver, Colorado

Enid Borden, CEO
Meals on Wheels Association of American Red Cross, Alexandria, Virginia

Trish Bunsen
Director, Senior Nutrition Sites, American Red Cross, Tacoma Pierce Chapter

Deborah Carmen, R.N., M.S.N.
Executive Advisor, Products and Health and Safety Services, American Red Cross National Headquarters

Mrs. Rosalynn Carter
Rosalynn Carter Institute for Caregiving,
Georgia Southwestern State University

Virginia L. Cheung, Attorney
Rockville, Maryland

Ron Coleman
Past President, International Association
of Fire Chiefs, Fairfax, Virginia

Ricky G. Davidson, M.D.
Boarded American Academy of Family
Physicians, Shreveport, Louisiana

**Jackie Gibbs, Fire Chief,
Marietta, Georgia**
Director, Fire and Life Safety Section,
International Association of Fire Chiefs,
Fairfax, Virginia

Elinor Ginzler
Director, Livable Communities, AARP
Office of Social Impact, Washington, D.C.

Mary T. Glenshaw, OT/L
Occupational Therapist, National
Rehabilitation Hospital, Washington, D.C.

Rick Greene, M.S.W.
Program Specialist, U.S. Administration
on Aging, Van Buren, Arkansas

Gail Gibson Hunt
Executive Director, National Alliance
for Caregiving, Bethesda, Maryland

Sally Hurme
Attorney, AARP Consumer Protection,
Washington, D.C.

Rhonda K. Hunter
Health Insurance Specialist, Centers
for Medicare and Medicaid Services

Vivian Littlefield, Ph.D., R.N., FAAN
National Chair of Nursing, American Red
Cross National Headquarters

Norma Olson, R.N.
Healthcare Programs, Senior Associate,
American Red Cross, Twin Cities Area
Chapter

Lydia Marien, M.S., A.R.N.P., B.C., F.N.P.
Family Nurse Practitioner and Volunteer,
American Red Cross, Greater Kansas City
Area Chapter

Nancy McKelvey, R.N., M.S.N.
Chief Nurse/Lead for Healthcare
Partnerships, American Red Cross
National Headquarters

Linda Morris, B.S.N., R.N.
Director, Community Health & Youth
Services, American Red Cross,
Greater Kansas City Area Chapter

Lin E. Noyes, Ph.D. R.N.
Clinical Director, Alzheimer's Family Day
Center, Falls Church, Virginia

Lisa Peters-Beumer, MPH
Project Director, Easter Seals,
Transportation Solutions for Caregivers

Charles P. Sabatino
Assistant Director, American Bar
Association, Commission on Law and Aging

Spencer Schron
Centers for Medicare and Medicaid
Services, (CMS-Central Office)

Lori Strauss
Coordinator, Benefits Outreach Program,
AARP Foundation, Washington, D.C.

Harry Wiland, M.F.A.
Executive Producer/Partner,
Wiland-Ball Productions, LLC

Table of Contents

Introduction

Perhaps former First Lady Rosalynn Carter said it best when she observed: "There are only four kinds of people in the world — those who *have been* caregivers, those who *currently are* caregivers, those who will be caregivers, and those who *will need* caregivers."

If you suddenly find yourself needing to know how to care for a loved one, you are not alone. About 50 million Americans care for a disabled, chronically ill or frail family member, and that number continues to grow as the U.S. population ages.

Whatever your circumstances, you can feel confident in having come to the right source for information about helping someone you love. The American Red Cross has been helping people learn how to take care of others for more than 100 years, and we want to help you, too. That's why we created this Family Caregiving book and its companion DVD. In this guide, you will find straightforward, trustworthy information thoroughly reviewed by American Red Cross nurses and other caregiving experts — all to make your caregiving role easier.

The book and DVD are designed to complement each other. As you read the book, you will notice special DVD icons in the margins. These indicate that the DVD contains more detailed information on that topic, or a demonstration of a specific skill. The DVD will show you in-depth how to perform caregiving skills more easily and safely in a step-by-step approach. To review a specific topic or skill, simply navigate to the chapter menu screen and scroll through the sub-menu to the topic you want.

The Red Cross is honored to have Mrs. Carter introduce the DVD. We hope you will listen to her advice to take good care of *yourself* — physically and emotionally — by accepting and seeking help from others. Caregivers often ignore their own needs when they care for someone they love. But by taking time for yourself, you will live a more balanced life and take even better care of your loved one.

In the end, you may find that despite the challenges, helping another person you care deeply about can result in personal fulfillment, spiritual growth and a deeper relationship with your loved one.

Best wishes on your journey,

Nancy McKelvey, MSN, R.N.
Chief Nurse
American Red Cross

Vivian Littlefield, PhD, R.N., FAAN
National Chair of Nursing (volunteer)
American Red Cross

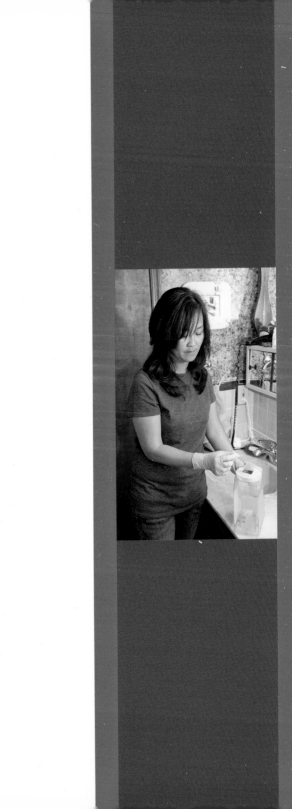

1

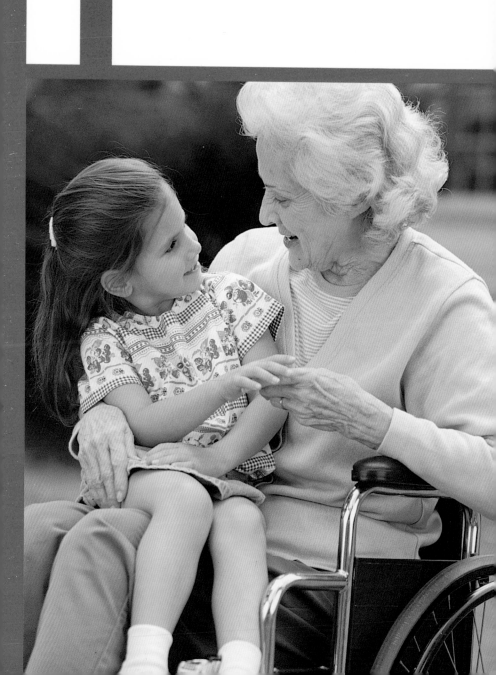

Home Safety

"I remember the day Mom was released from the hospital," recalls Gwen. "Besides her mobility problems, the stroke left Mom a little confused and with impaired vision — especially on her left side. Before she came to live with us we had to do a room-to-room safety sweep. We removed clutter and throw rugs, rearranged furniture and installed grab bars in the shower. We told the children they would have to be very diligent about picking up their things so Grandma wouldn't trip. The kids even took turns scooting around the house in her wheelchair to see if there were any obstacles we overlooked."

tips

Reduce Hazards in Your Home

Remove clutter and obstacles:

☐ Remove tripping hazards such as electrical cords, papers, books and shoes from floors and stairs.

☐ Make sure there is a clear path around furniture.

Stairs and hallways:

☐ Keep stairs and hallways well lit and clutter-free.

☐ Install sturdy, well-secured handrails on both sides of stairs and hallways.

☐ Make sure your loved one wears slippers or shoes with nonskid soles when using stairs. Socks or smooth-soled slippers or shoes may cause her to slip and fall.

Provide a Safe Environment

To help an elderly loved one maintain her independence, make the home environment as safe as possible. Use common sense and your knowledge of your loved one to anticipate things that could go wrong, then take steps to prevent them.

Inspect each room for potential safety hazards. If your loved one is wheelchair-bound, get down on her level. If you notice a safety threat, correct it right away if possible.

Prevent Falls

Falls are a leading cause of injuries, hospitalizations and deaths among the elderly. The majority of falls happen in the home. If your loved one is weak, confused or unsteady on her feet, she is more likely to fall or injure herself. Help prevent falls by following these guidelines:

• Attend to health issues that increase your loved one's risk of falls.

- Maintain a regular exercise program. Exercise improves strength, balance and coordination.
- Have the health-care provider review your loved one's medicines (both prescription and over-the-counter) to reduce side effects and avoid drug interactions.
- Have your loved one's vision checked annually. Poor vision can increase the risk of falling. If your loved one wears eyeglasses, make sure they are clean.
- To prevent your loved one from falling out of bed, use guardrails and position her in the middle of the bed so she can turn over safely.

Electrical Safety
Extension cords are not intended for long-term use.

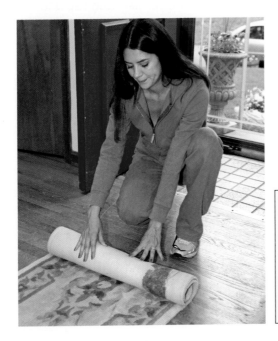

Remove throw rugs, which can slip, or secure them with double-sided tape or rubber nonskid matting.

tips

Reduce Hazards in Your Home

Focus on flooring:
- [ ] Remove throw rugs, which can slip, or secure them with double-sided tape or rubber nonskid matting.
- [ ] Tack down edges of carpets and repair, replace or remove carpeting that is worn, torn or frayed.
- [ ] Keep floors dry. Wipe up spills immediately, and follow infection control procedures when necessary. (See Body Fluid Cleanup on page 12)
- [ ] Use nonwax cleaning products on floors.

If an extension cord is needed for longer than 1 day, have an additional electrical outlet installed.

Do not tuck an extension cord under a rug. Secure it to the wall or floor with tape or commercial products made to hide the cords. Never leave extension cords lying loosely on the floor or hanging across a pathway.

Do not overload extension cords or electrical circuits. Unplug electrical equipment when not in use and replace frayed cords.

Telephone Access
Make sure your loved one can call for help in an emergency. Place at least one telephone where it can be reached in case your loved one is unable to stand and move around.

If your loved one wears a hearing aid, make sure it works and encourage her to use it.

Post emergency phone numbers near each phone in the house. Be sure to include

Equipment Safety

Caring for a loved one at home can involve unfamiliar equipment, such as a wheelchair, walker or hospital bed. Before using any piece of equipment, take the time to understand how it works by reading the product manual and following instructions exactly. Improper use can cause serious injuries. (If no manual is available, you may find instructions on a sticker or label attached to the equipment.) You may also ask the health-care provider, a home health nurse or equipment retailer to teach you how to use the equipment.

Before using the equipment with your loved one, practice the correct procedure by yourself.

Use Brakes. The brakes provided on wheeled equipment — beds, wheelchairs, shower chairs — prevent unwanted rolling. Test the brakes before using a piece of

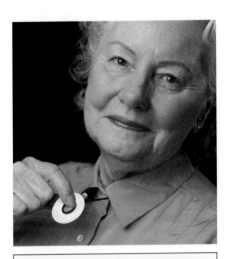

Contract with a medical alert service, such as LifeLine,® so your loved one can summon help if she can't get to a telephone.

the National Poison Control number: 800-222-1222. Post your phone number on each telephone in the house. Also, post the street names of the nearest intersection near each phone.

Have a cell phone available for emergency use, if possible.

wheeled equipment. Make sure they work properly. If they do not, do not use the equipment.

Before helping your loved one into or out of a wheelchair, lock the brakes and make sure the chair is secure. Also, before stepping away from someone in a wheelchair, make sure both wheelchair brakes are locked securely.

Fire Safety

Do not let your loved one smoke unsupervised. Keep candles away from combustible materials and do not leave your loved one unattended in a room with lit candles.

Do not overload electrical outlets or use appliances with frayed or cracked wires.

Label shut-off valves for

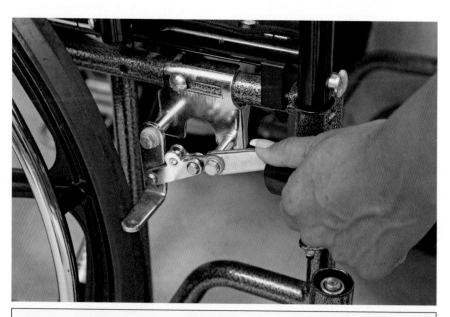

Test the brakes before using a piece of wheeled equipment. Make sure they work properly.

gas, oil, water and electricity.

Schedule Routine Inspections

Inspect fireplaces, fuel-burning heaters and woodstoves. Have chimney connections and flues inspected by a professional and cleaned, if necessary, before every heating season.

Make sure they are properly vented to the outside to prevent carbon monoxide poisoning.

Alarms and Fire Extinguishers

Test your smoke and fire detectors every month to make sure they work properly.

Have one or more working fire extinguishers in your home and know how to use them properly.

Change the batteries and examine your fire extinguisher and detectors twice a year when you change the clocks.

tips

Reduce Hazards in Your Home

Reduce bathroom hazards:

☐ Make sure tubs and showers have a textured surface or nonskid mats or strips both inside and on the floor outside.

☐ Install grab bars in the tub, shower and by the toilet for support.

☐ Use a shower chair and a handheld showerhead to make bathing safer and easier.

☐ Check the water temperature with a bath thermometer or the back of your hand before your loved one enters the tub or shower. Turn hot water on last and off first. Set the hot water heater to low or no higher than 108° F.

tips

Reduce Hazards in Your Home

Improve lighting visibility:

- ☐ Make sure your home is well lit (use at least 60-watt bulbs; frosted light-bulbs reduce glare).
- ☐ Install nightlights in your loved one's bedroom, bathroom and hallway and at the top and bottom of stairways.
- ☐ Use reflective tape at the top and bottom of stairs.

Portable Space Heaters

Place space heaters at least 3 feet away from pets, people and anything combustible.

Never leave space heaters on when you are not in the room or when you go to bed.

If you have a fuel-burning space heater and people in the room begin to have nausea, vomiting, a headache or begin to feel sick, turn off the heater and get fresh air immediately.

Cooking Safety

When cooking, do not wear loose-fitting clothing or clothing with dangling sleeves. Always turn pot handles inward.

Oxygen Safety

If your loved one's health-care provider recommends extra oxygen to help her breathe, ask the health-care provider for the correct oxygen flow rate and when to change it. Your loved one's health-care provider will tell you if and when to adjust the flow rate.

If your loved one uses supplemental oxygen, take precautions to make sure it is safe. Keep oxygen away from open flames or high heat. This includes cigarette smoke, radiators or space heaters and some electrical appliances, particularly electric shavers.

Keep all flammable items such as aerosol sprays, alcohol, gasoline, perfume and wool clothing away from the oxygen supply.

Keep oxygen tanks in a stable position to prevent them from falling over.

Have a backup oxygen supply plan in case the tank runs empty after business hours or during weekends and holidays. If your loved one uses an elec-

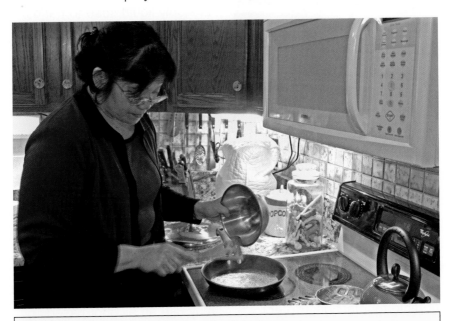

When cooking, do not wear loose-fitting clothing or clothing with dangling sleeves and always turn pot handles inward.

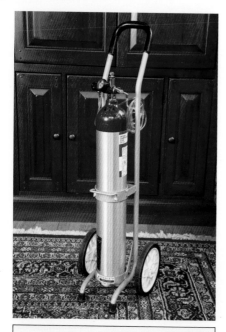

Follow the oxygen supplier's instructions for safe storage and equipment use.

tric oxygen machine, learn how to administer oxygen manually in case the electricity goes out.

Infection Control

Your loved one may be vulnerable to infection. Protect yourself and your loved one by treating all blood and body fluids as if they are infectious and wash hands often to remove bacteria and viruses that can cause disease. Also, use a disinfectant cleaner on household surfaces.

Washing Hands
To wash your hands correctly:
1. Wet hands with warm, running water.
2. Apply liquid soap to hands.
3. Rub hands vigorously for at least 15 seconds, covering all surfaces of the hands and fingers including fingernails and around jewelry. Scrub nails by rubbing them against the palms of your hands.
4. Rinse hands with water.
5. Dry hands thoroughly with a paper towel.
6. Use the paper towel to turn off the faucet.

If hands do not look dirty, you may use an alcohol-based hand sanitizer instead of, or in addition to, washing.

⊚ Disposable Gloves

Another precaution is to wear disposable gloves when you perform these tasks:

- When in contact with your loved one's semen, vaginal fluid, cuts, sores, blood or other body fluids such as urine, feces or vomit.
- When providing care to your loved one's mouth, rectum or genitals.
- When changing diapers or sanitary pads or to empty bedpans or urinals.
- If you have cuts, sores, rashes or breaks in your own skin, cover them with a bandage and wear disposable gloves.

You can purchase disposable gloves at most drugstores. Use the gloves only once, then throw them away. Do not use gloves more than one time even if they are marked "reusable."

In some cases insurance companies and Medicaid will

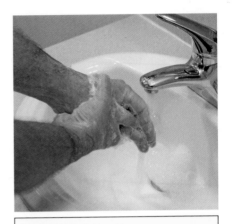

Wash hands with liquid soap and warm running water.

pay for disposable gloves if the health-care provider writes a prescription for them.

Disposable gloves are available in latex, vinyl or nitrile. Some people are sensitive to latex and may have an allergic reaction to it. Symptoms include skin redness, rash, hives, itching, runny nose, sneezing, itchy eyes, scratchy throat or shortness of breath.

If you experience any of these symptoms, remove gloves and wash your hands immediately. If conditions persist or if you experience a severe reaction, get medical attention right away.

Body Fluid Cleanup

Because viruses and bacteria can be found in semen, vaginal fluid, feces, breast milk or blood, clean up these spills quickly.

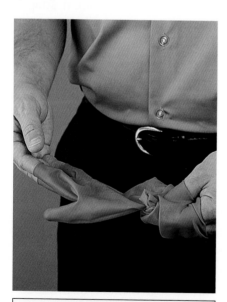

Touch only the interior surfaces when removing disposable gloves

Put on gloves, wipe up the fluid with paper towels or rags, put the used paper towels or rags in plastic bags to dispose of later, then wipe the area clean with a fresh mixture of ¼ cup bleach per gallon of water. Allow the solution to stand on the surface for at least 10 minutes or allow the surface to air dry.

If you get body fluid in your eyes, nose, mouth, or a cut or open wound, immediately flush the affected area with water, call the health-care provider, explain what happened and ask what else you should do.

In some cases, appropriate barriers such as dust/particulate mask and/or eye shields may be necessary. Consult your health-care provider for guidance on appropriate personal protective equipment or special hand-washing and cleanup procedures for your situation.

Needles and Syringes

Your loved one may need needles and syringes to take medicine. If you handle these, be careful not to stick yourself.

Use a needle and syringe only once and do not put caps back on needles. Most needle-stick injuries occur when recapping is attempted. Do not take needles off syringes, or bend or break needles.

If a needle falls off a syringe, use tweezers or pliers to pick it up — do not use your fingers.

Touch needles and syringes only by the barrel of the syringe and always hold the sharp end away from you.

Put the used needle and syringe in a puncture-proof container, such as a coffee can or glass bottle. You can also get a special container from the health-care provider or nurse. Keep containers in the rooms where needles and syringes are used.

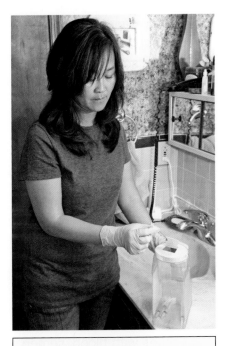

Put used needles and syringes in a puncture-proof container.

Ask the health-care provider or nurse how to get rid of the container with used needles and syringes.

If you get stuck with a used needle:

- Put the needle in the used-needle container.

- Wash the stuck area with warm, soapy water, and use a circular scrubbing motion.
- Call your health-care provider or the emergency room, explain what happened and ask what else you should do. You may be advised to take medicine for post-exposure treatment.

Dispose of Waste Safely

Always wear disposable gloves and flush down the toilet all liquid waste such as urine and vomit as well as toilet paper and tissues with blood, semen, vaginal fluid or breast milk. Be careful to not splash when you pour liquids into the toilet.

Place paper towels, sanitary pads, diapers, bandages and other items that cannot be flushed in a closed and sealed plastic bag. Ask the health-care provider, nurse or local health department how to get rid of items with body fluids on them.

Medication Safety

It is important to keep a comprehensive list of your loved one's medications (including dose and frequency of prescriptions, over-the-counter medications and herbal supplements). (See insert on page 124.) Copy this list and post a copy on the refrigerator, near telephones, and have your loved one keep a copy in her purse or wallet.

Bring the list with you when taking your loved one to the doctor, pharmacist, hospital or other health-care provider. Doing so will help professional caregivers ensure that she receives appropriate medical care.

Store all medicines and cleaning materials in locked cabinets and closets.

Emergency Preparedness

It is more important than ever that you be prepared for possible disasters and other emergencies. Natural or human-caused disasters can strike suddenly, at anytime and anywhere. There are **three actions** everyone can take that can help make a difference...

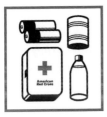

1. Get a Kit

What you have on hand when a disaster happens can make a big difference. Have at least 3 days of supplies in an easy-to-carry evacuation kit, with additional supplies at home in case you cannot leave.

Remember to check your kit and replace the stock every 6 months.

An easy way to get your kit started is to contact your local Red Cross chapter or go online at **www.redcross.org** to order your emergency preparedness kit today. If you purchase a kit or choose to build your own, check that it includes the following:

Water. Include at least one gallon per person per day.
Food. Include non-perishable foods you enjoy that require no refrigeration, preparation or cooking and little or no water. This may include high-protein items, including energy bars, ready-to-eat soup, peanut butter, etc.
Flashlight. Include extra batteries, or use an alternate energy option.
First aid kit. Include a first aid reference guide.
Medications. Remember to include prescription and non-prescription medications, and copies of the prescriptions.
Radio. Include batteries or use an alternate energy option.
Tools. Include a wrench, a manual can opener, screwdriver, hammer, pliers, knife, duct tape, plastic sheeting and garbage bags.

Clothing. Have a change of clothes for everyone, including sturdy shoes and work gloves.
Personal items. Eyeglasses or contact lenses and solution; unique items for infants, seniors and people with disabilities.
Copies of important papers. Include identification cards, insurance policies, birth certificates, passports, etc.

Comfort items. Include some toys and books.
Sanitary supplies. Toilet paper, towelettes, feminine supplies, personal hygiene items, bleach, etc.
Money. Cash and coins in case credit cards do not work.
Contact list. Include family phone numbers, e-mail addresses, meeting locations and out-of-

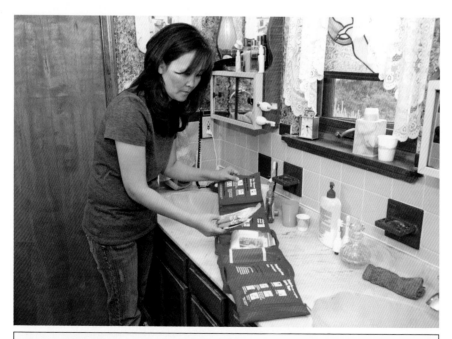

It's important to have a well-stocked first aid kit.

area contact information.

Pet supplies. Food, water, leash, litter box or plastic bags, tags, medications and vaccination information.

Map. Mark this with evacuation routes from your local area.

Store your disaster supplies in sturdy yet easy-to-carry containers. Keep a smaller version of the kit in your vehicle. If you become stranded, or are not able to return home, having some items with you may keep you more comfortable until help arrives.

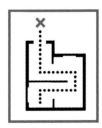

2. Make a Plan

Planning ahead is the first step to a more calm and assured disaster response.

Talk. Discuss with your family the disasters that can happen where you live. Establish responsibilities for each member of your household and plan to work together as a team. Designate alternates in case someone is absent. If a family member is in the military, also plan for how you would respond if they are deployed and include the local military base resources that may be available.

Plan. Choose two places to meet after a disaster:
- Right outside your home, in case of a sudden emergency, such as a fire.
- Outside your neighborhood, in case you cannot return home or are asked to evacuate your neighborhood.

Learn. Each adult in your household should learn how and when to turn off utilities such as electricity, water and gas. Ask someone at your local fire department to show you how to use a fire extinguisher.

Tell. Everyone in the household should know where emergency information and supplies are kept. Make copies for everyone to carry with them. Keep the information updated.

Practice. Evacuate your home twice a year. Drive your planned evacuation route and plot alternate routes on a map in case main roads are impassable or gridlocked.

Include your pets. If you must evacuate, take your animals with you. If it is not safe for you, it is not safe for them.

Support your community. Some caregivers feel that they get a welcome break by taking a little time to help others in their communities. Support your community by volunteering and by giving blood.

More than one million Americans serve their communities as volunteers. Red Cross volunteers help people in emergencies; they teach first aid classes; organize blood drives; and translate so that non-English speakers can receive Red Cross services. They connect members of the armed forces stationed overseas with their families.

Blood is needed in times of emergency, but the ongoing need is also great. Every two seconds someone needs a blood transfusion — cancer patients, accident victims, premature infants, people with chronic diseases.

Giving blood doesn't take much time. During times of crisis and every day, each blood donation has the power to help save as many as 3 lives.

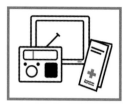

3. Be Informed

Knowing what may happen and how you can help can make all the difference when an emergency happens.

Learn what disasters or emergencies may occur where you live, work and play. These events can vary from impacting only you and your family — such as a home fire or medical emergency — or your entire community — such as an earthquake or flood. **Find out how local authorities will notify you** during a disaster and how you will get important information, including local radio, TV and NOAA weather radio.

Learn what you can do to prepare for these events by contacting your local Red Cross chapter to ask about first aid and CPR, and disaster training.

Learning simple first aid techniques can give you the

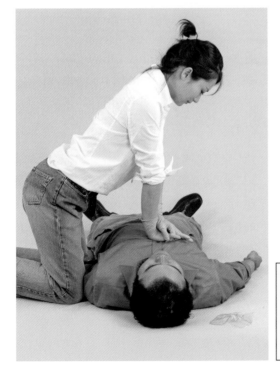

Make sure that at least one member of your household is trained in first aid and CPR.

skills and confidence to help anyone in your home, your neighborhood and at work.

When a major disaster occurs, your community can change in an instant. Loved ones can be hurt and emergency response can be delayed. Make sure that at least one member of your household is trained in first aid and CPR and in how to use an automated external defibrillator (AED).

Disaster preparedness presentations will provide more specific information on how to prepare for disasters in your community. Contact your local American Red Cross chapter for details.

The 3 steps below can help you to react well in an emergency:

- **Check the scene** for safety and the person for life-threatening conditions.
- **Call 9-1-1** or your local emergency number and request professional assistance.
- **Care for the person** if you can reach him safely.

Share what you have learned with your family, household and neighbors and encourage them to be informed too.

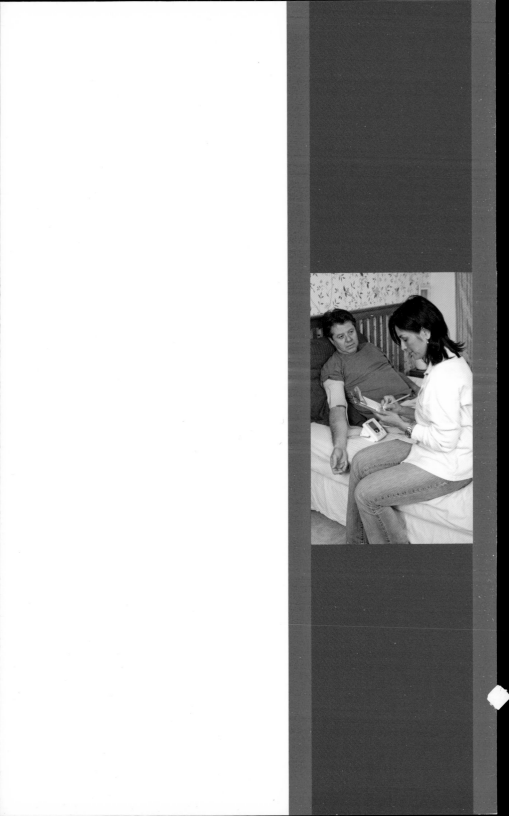

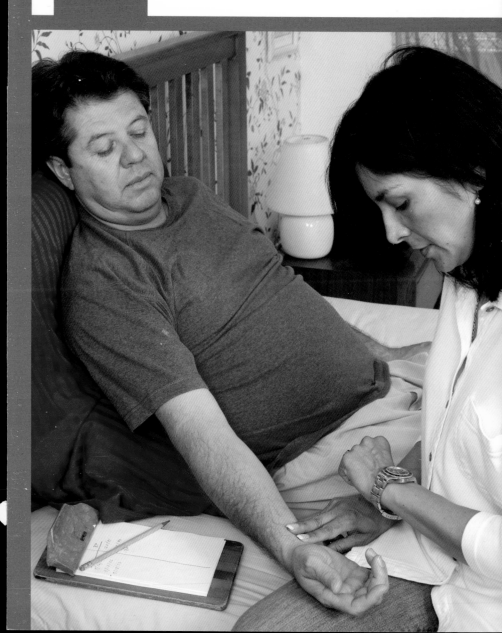

2

Caregiving Skills

"I called the doctor whenever Jack's breathing suddenly became more labored than usual," says Donna, as she recalls caregiving for Jack, her late husband. "The doctor always asked me about Jack's body temperature, pulse, respiration rate and what he had eaten and when. After Jack's diagnosis with cancer, the doctor said I should call him right away if Jack was fighting off an infection or had indigestion or food poisoning."

tips

Keep A Vital Signs Notebook

A health-care provider may suggest keeping a record of your loved one's vital signs to help him or her monitor your loved one's health.

Take vital signs at about the same time each day and evening. Record the date, time, temperature, pulse, respiration and blood pressure.

Vital sign readings may show physical changes that occur when the body is fighting an infection or disease. Some of the first changes may be a rise in body temperature and a faster heartbeat and breathing rate.

◎ Reading and Recording Vital Signs

Chances are you and your health-care provider won't be able to tell how your loved one's body is functioning by only his appearance, although that will give you clues. You have to read the signs — the vital signs: pulse, breathing rate, blood pressure and temperature — to know how the body is working.

Your loved one's health-care provider may recommend that you or a home health aide measure your loved one's vital signs when his condition changes. This will also help the health-care provider decide what treatment or medication your loved one should receive.

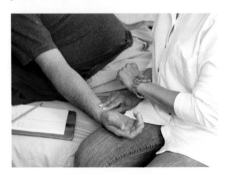

What Vital Signs Measure

Body temperature is the amount of heat in the body.

Breathing rate is how fast air moves in and out of the lungs per minute. One respiration is one inhalation plus one exhalation.

Pulse is how fast the heart is beating.

Blood pressure is the force exerted against the blood vessels (arteries) when the heart pumps blood.

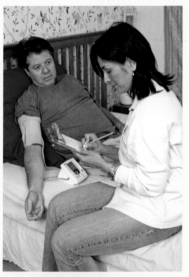

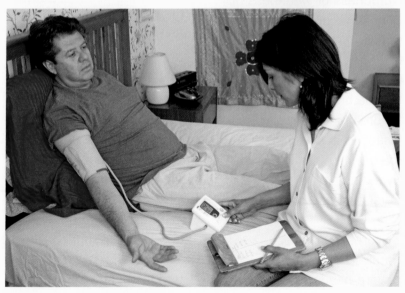

Sudden Illness

When a person becomes suddenly ill, he or she usually looks and feels sick. **CALL 9-1-1** or your local emergency number if your loved one has any of the following signals:

- Changes in consciousness (such as feeling lightheaded, dizzy or becoming unconscious)
- Nausea or vomiting
- Difficulty speaking or slurred speech
- Numbness or weakness
- Loss of vision, or blurred vision
- Changes in breathing (The person may have trouble breathing or may not be breathing normally.)
- Changes in skin color (pale, ashen or flushed skin)
- Sweating
- Persistent pressure or pain
- Diarrhea
- Seizures
- Paralysis or inability to move
- Severe headache

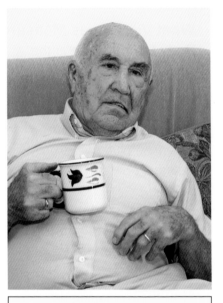

One of the primary signals of a stroke is sudden facial drooping or weakness on one side of the face.

In many cases, receiving prompt care can ensure a positive outcome to the medical emergency.

Stroke: What to Look For
As with other sudden illnesses, the primary signals are a sudden change in how the

body is working or feeling:

- Sudden body weakness or numbness, often on one side of the body
- Sudden facial drooping or weakness on one side of the face
- Trouble speaking or being understood when speaking
- Has blurred or dimmed vision
- Sudden severe headache
- Dizziness or confusion

If you notice your loved one is having or has had a stroke:

- Send someone to **CALL 9-1-1** or the local emergency number immediately.
- If the person is drooling or having difficulty swallowing, place him on his side to keep the airway clear.

The F.A.S.T. mnemonic in the sidebar on the right is based on the Cincinnati Pre-Hospital Stroke Scale to help identify if a person has experienced a stroke.

For a Stroke, Think F.A.S.T.

FACE – Weakness on one side of the face
Ask the person to smile; this will show if there is drooping or weakness in the muscles on one side of the face.

ARM – Weakness or numbness in one arm
Ask the person to raise both arms to find out if there is weakness in one limb (both arms will not be raised to same level).

SPEECH – Slurred speech or trouble getting the words out
Ask the person to say a simple sentence or phrase and listen for slurred or distorted speech (e.g. "Mary had a little lamb").

TIME – Time to CALL 9-1-1 if you see any of these signs
If the person has difficulty with any of these tasks, or shows other signals of a stroke, note the time that the signals began and **CALL 9-1-1** right away.

Giving Medication

Your loved one may be taking prescription medicine as well as over-the-counter (OTC) medicines and food supplements. OTC medicine can include vitamins, laxatives, cold medicines, herbal remedies and antacids.

Both prescription and OTC medicine can cause serious problems if not taken correctly. Be very careful to give medications exactly the way the health-care provider advises.

To be safe, don't change medication dosage without first checking with the health-care provider.

You and your loved one should learn about the medicines he takes and know when to take them and their possible side effects.

Some questions to ask
- What is the medicine's name?
- Why is my loved one taking

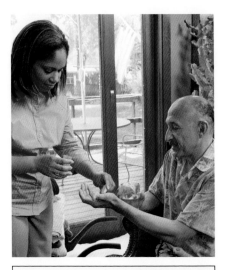

Be careful to give medications exactly the way the health-care provider advises.

this medicine?
- Should my loved one take this medicine on an empty stomach or with food?
- If I forget to give my loved one a dose of the medicine, what should I do?
- How much should I give him?
- How long should he take it?
- What problems should I watch for?

Do's and Don'ts of Medicine

DO let your health-care provider know if you think the medicine is working.

DO always tell the health-care provider about past problems your loved one has had with drugs, such as rashes, indigestion or dizziness.

DO call the health-care provider right away if your loved one has any problems with the medicine.

DO make sure that the health-care provider knows all of the medicines that your loved one is taking before he advises you to either stop a medicine or start a new one.

DO store oral medications separate from other medications — such as lotions, eye-drops and suppositories.

DON'T mix alcohol and medicine unless the health-care provider says it is OK. Some drugs may not work well or may make your loved one sick if taken with alcohol.

DON'T crush or chew tablets or pills unless the health-care provider or pharmacist says it is OK.

DON'T have your loved one "make up" a dose if he misses one unless advised to do so by the health-care provider.

DON'T give your loved one medicine prescribed for another person.

DON'T give any medicine to your loved one without the health-care provider's approval.

Your Pharmacy Can Help

Pharmacists are a great resource for medication questions. Try to use the same pharmacy for all prescriptions and OTC medicines. That way, the pharmacist will be able to advise you about potential medication interactions. Ask the pharmacist to add OTC medications, herbal remedies and any mail order prescriptions to the file.

Keep Medication Records

As a caregiver, you may be faced with a complicated medication schedule. Because it is so important that correct medicine be taken at the correct times, it helps to keep records of all medicine being taken. If your loved one becomes seriously ill, keeping records becomes even more important.

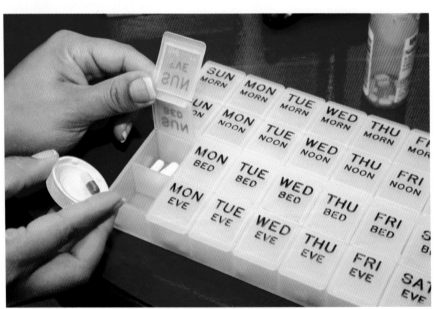

This kind of container can help you remember to give each dose.

Remember these 5 RIGHTS to giving medication

Right Person: Give medication only to the person for whom it is prescribed.

Right Time: Give the medication at the time of day and frequency the doctor prescribed.

Right Medication: The person in your care may have to take several medications a day. Read the label to ensure that you are giving the correct one.

Right Amount: Give only the prescribed amount.

Right Route: Medications come in many forms; some may be for oral use, others are to be used only in the nose or on the skin. Note how the medication is to be given.

Keep a medications list for your loved one that includes the names of the medication, prescription number, who prescribed it and why, amount and when taken and special directions for its use or precautions to follow. Take this list with you when you go to the health-care provider.

You may also find that daily or weekly medicine containers (available at most drugstores) help you and your loved one remember to take each dose.

Read the Label

Read the label before giving any medication. If the label is hard to read, ask your pharmacist to use larger type or keep a bright light and a magnifying glass handy for reading labels. The label should show:

- **List of Ingredients.** If you know your loved one is allergic to anything in the medicine, don't use it. Ask the health-care provider or pharmacist for a different medicine.

- **Warnings.** Read these carefully.
- **The Expiration Date.** Do not use a medicine after the expiration date on the container.
- **Side Effects.** Some medicines can cause problems, or side effects. Side effects may include sleepiness, vomiting, bleeding, headaches or rashes. Ask about the side effects of the medicine your loved one is taking. Talk about them with the health-care provider, pharmacist or nurse.

Avoid Problems

Organize your loved one's medicine. Your loved one should not "make up" a dose if he misses one unless advised to do so by the health-care provider. Do not share medicines, and keep a list of the medicines your loved one takes.

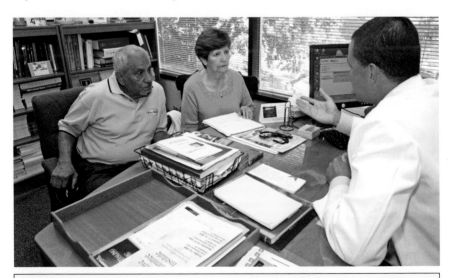

Make sure you understand the information your loved one's health-care provider or home health nurse gives you.

Communication and Organization

Although it may sometimes feel like it, you are not alone in providing care for your loved one. His health-care professionals are there to help. Think of them as part of your caregiving team and do not hesitate to call them and ask questions.

It is important that you communicate with your loved one's health-care professionals about his condition and the care you provide. Here are some tips:

- Make sure you understand the information your loved one's health-care provider or home health nurse gives you. Ask a lot of questions and keep asking until you get the answers you need.
- Have a list of questions ready and write down the answers. Do not trust this to your memory alone.
- Keep your loved one's medical information in front of you when talking with his health-care provider or home health nurse.

Time-Saving Ideas

These helpful tips will help you get more done in a day, but don't pressure yourself to do too much for your loved one. Plan to take time for yourself too.

Organize Supplies

Organize the supplies you need for your loved one's morning and bedtime routines (e.g., medication, personal items, clothing), and keep them well stocked and in your loved one's room for easy access.

Get Help

If your loved one needs a lot of assistance (morning and bedtime routines will usually take the most time), ask a friend, family member or home health aide for help.

Do not try to do everything by yourself and don't wait for someone else to offer to help

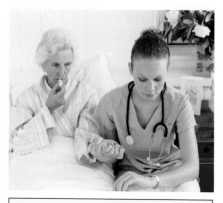

If your loved one needs a lot of assistance, ask a friend, family member or home health aide for help.

— ask! For example, if you are caring for your mother, ask a sibling to sit with her each Saturday morning for 2 hours while you take a break.

Simplify the Laundry
Instead of ironing your loved one's clothes, try putting them in a dryer with a wet towel. You'll be amazed at how few wrinkles there are.

Use a water-resistant mattress pad under regular sheets on your loved one's bed if she is incontinent. This will help protect the mattress. Also use a disposable bed protector under your loved one to keep the sheets cleaner longer.

Choose Easy Clothes
Loose-fitting pants with elastic or drawstring waistbands are easier to put on and take off.

Shirts that snap or zipper down the front are much easier to put on than button-down shirts or pullovers.

Shoes that have Velcro® fasteners or zippers are easier to put on and take off than shoes with laces.

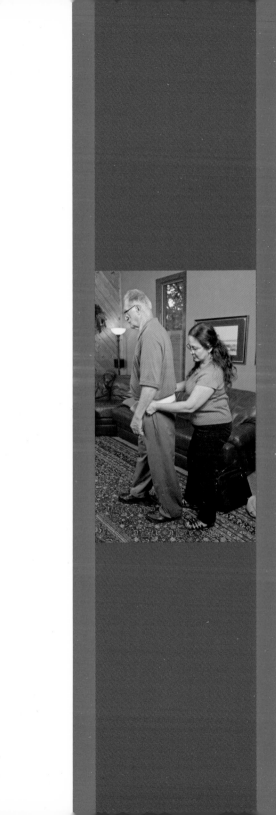

3

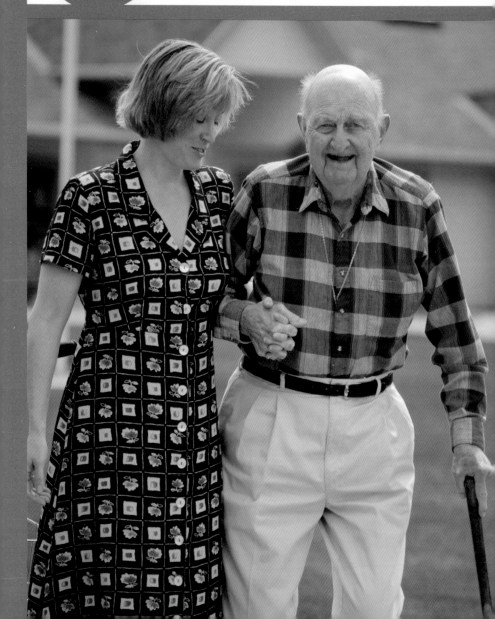

Body Mechanics

"After the stroke, Dad's physical therapist told us it was important for him to use his walker several times every day to help his brain relearn how to walk," recalls Cindi. "But getting him out of the bed or wheelchair was a real project. My husband Chris and I worked together to help him. Othewise Dad and I both might have landed on the floor."

tips

How to Prevent Muscle, Joint and Back Strain

- ☐ Wear proper footwear. Use comfortable, well-fitted, low-heeled shoes with nonskid soles.
- ☐ Exercise regularly. Exercise can increase blood circulation and strengthen muscles.
- ☐ Use good posture. Sit or stand up straight with your shoulders centered over your hips.
- ☐ Place frequently used objects within arm's reach. Store these items between knuckle and shoulder height.

◎ Prevent Strains

While helping your loved one, be aware of protecting your own muscles and joints. Each time you lift, push, pull or twist your body, you increase your risk of back injury. Apply the principles of good body mechanics to protect yourself from injury.

Keep Moving

Activity is important because it strengthens muscles and improves blood flow and mental attitude. It also helps maintain regular bowel movements and can help a person sleep better.

Prevent Pressure Ulcers

Moving around is especially important for a person who is unable to get out of bed. Changing positions in bed can help prevent pressure ulcers, also called bedsores. Pressure ulcers are caused by anything that rubs or presses against the skin for a period of time, such as a mattress or wrinkled sheets.

Pressure ulcers are difficult to heal. That's why prevention is extremely important.

In people with light skin, pressure ulcers first appear as red and tender areas of the skin. In people with dark skin, the first sign of a pressure ulcer is an area of the skin that is darker than normal. These stressed areas of the skin then break down into sores, and are most likely to occur on bony areas of the body such as elbows, shoulders, heels and the tailbone.

Pressure ulcers can develop rapidly. The best way to prevent them is to make sure your loved one changes position at least every 2 hours. Be sure to relieve the pressure points she was lying on. For example, if

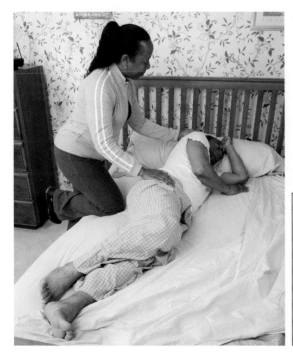

Pressure ulcers can develop rapidly. To prevent them, make sure your loved one changes position at least every 2 hours.

tips

How to Prevent Muscle, Joint and Back Strain

- ☐ Avoid reaching across an extended space. As you lift a heavy object or move your loved one, keep her close to your body.
- ☐ Push and pull heavy objects or your loved one, if possible, instead of lifting. Lifting can cause greater strain on your back and muscles.

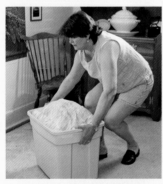

- ☐ Bend at the knees and hips when lifting heavy objects. Do not bend at the waist.

your loved one is lying on her back with the head of the bed raised, then reposition her on her side. When she is on her back, the shoulder blades, heels and elbows are under pressure. When her position changes to the side, then her ear, shoulder, hip, knee and ankle receive pressure. Later, have her change to the other side.

By paying attention to where your loved one's body comes into contact with the bed, you can make sure she does not lie on one spot for too long.

Positioning Your Loved One in Bed

Make sure your loved one's bones and joints are in a natural position that feels comfortable. Support the bones and joints to minimize strain on them. For example, you could place a small pillow under the calves to lift the heels away from the mattress and relieve pressure.

Encourage your loved one to

10 Ways to Prevent Pressure Ulcers

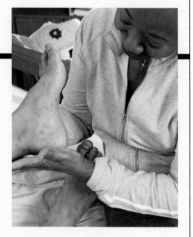

1. Keep your loved one's skin clean and dry.
2. Check daily for changes in skin color under breasts, skin folds and on bony prominences.
3. Avoid friction when moving or positioning your loved one. You may need help to do this.
4. Gently massage the skin around pressure areas (e.g., elbows, shoulders, heels, tailbone) with a circular motion to promote circulation.
5. Help your loved one reposition herself every 2 hours.
6. Keep your loved one's bed as wrinkle-free as possible.
7. Use a padded mattress and an egg crate or sheepskin mattress pad, available at medical supply stores.
8. Encourage your loved one to drink plenty of fluids.
9. Provide a well-balanced diet. A high protein diet promotes healing. Check with the health-care provider before initiating a high protein diet, because people with certain health problems, such as renal disease (kidney disease), should not receive a high protein diet.
10. Encourage or assist your loved one to get out of bed regularly, if possible.

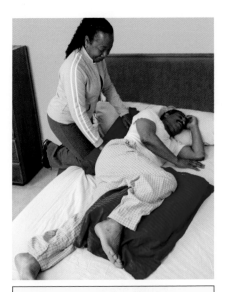

Adding supports will help keep your loved one in the proper position.

move around as much as he can on his own to maintain his independence. As you prepare to help, explain what you are doing so that he may assist you if possible. Work together to help both of you prevent injuries.

Range of Motion Exercises
Ask your loved one's health-care provider or physical therapist what range of motion exercises are appropriate for him. Arm, leg and foot exercises help prevent stiff, sore joints and improve circulation. If your loved one is unable to do exercises himself, you can do them for him by moving his joints.

Positioning Your Loved One on the Side
Moving your loved one frequently to help prevent pressure ulcers and improve circulation may mean that you have to change his position from on his back to on his side. Follow these steps:

1. If possible, have your loved one cross his arms over his chest and cross his ankles toward the direction you are turning him.
2. Put your hand on your loved one's shoulder and the other on his upper thigh.
3. Roll your loved one onto his side toward you.
4. Adjust your loved one's

shoulder so that he is not lying on his arm.

5. Support your loved one's back with a rolled blanket, towel or pillow folded in half, to keep him in proper position.
6. Support his top arm with a pillow.
7. Place his top leg forward and place a pillow between his legs so that it does not rest directly on top of the lower leg.

Sitting on the Edge of the Bed

Before your loved one gets up and out of bed, it is a good idea for him to sit on the edge of the bed for a few minutes to get his balance and acclimate his blood pressure. Encourage him to do as much as he can on his own.

1. Slowly and gently help him sit up in bed.
2. Help him scoot his body to the edge of the bed.
3. Gently swing his legs over the side of the bed.
4. Have him stay seated for a few minutes before standing or moving to a chair or wheelchair.

Getting from the Bed to a Chair

1. Place the wheelchair or stationary chair at a slight angle at the head of the bed on the person's stronger side.
2. Lock the bed brakes, if applicable. If a wheelchair is used, fold back the footrests and lock the brakes.
3. Help your loved one put on nonskid slippers or footwear.
4. Turn him toward you into a sitting position so that his legs dangle over the side of the bed.

Note: Stay with your loved one and encourage him to sit on the side of the bed for a few minutes before continuing. Some dizziness is common when a person

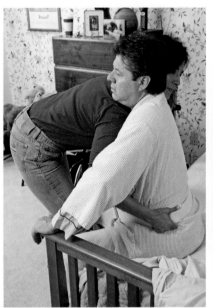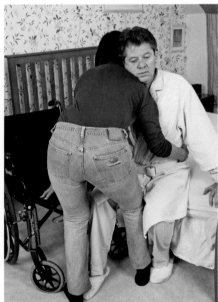

Securely grip your loved one's waistband. Stagger your feet by placing one foot facing your loved one with your knee between his knees and your other foot farther back.

sits up after being in bed for a while. If it doesn't pass, gets worse, if he becomes sweaty, short of breath or if he is in any pain, have him lie back down.

5. Securely grip your loved one's waistband. When your loved one gets ready to move, his buttocks should be at the edge of the bed and he should be leaning slightly forward. His feet should be flat on the floor with toes pointed straight ahead. If the chair he will move to is on your left, place your right foot

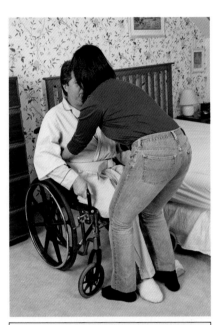

Lower your loved one into the chair by bending your knees and keeping your back straight.

of injury for short distance transfers from or to a bed, chair, toilet or car. It can also be used to help support a person during walking.

6. Have your loved one use his hands to push himself up, if possible. Encourage him to help as much as he can.

7. Stagger your feet by placing one foot facing your loved one with your knee (the one farthest from the chair) between his knees and your other foot farther back. Keep both feet facing your loved one. Bend your knees, tighten your abdominal and buttocks muscles and keep your back straight.

8. Tell your loved one that on the count of three you are going to help him into the chair. Rock back and forth gently on each count to create momentum and, on the count of three, help him to move up and over. Keep

between his feet.

Note: Talk with your loved one's doctor or physical therapist about the various assistive devices that can make caring for your loved one easier and safer. For example, a gait or transfer belt can help reduce the risk

tips

Moving to a Chair

- ☐ Get as close as possible in a "hugging" position.
- ☐ Use a good base of support.
- ☐ Keep the person close.
- ☐ Keep your back straight.
- ☐ Lift smoothly. Do not jerk or twist.
- ☐ Put your head to your loved one's side closest to the chair so you can keep the chair in sight during the move.

him close as you straighten your legs. Turn your body and your loved one's together as you pivot him until he is right in front of the wheelchair.

9. Lower your loved one into the chair by bending your knees and keeping your back straight. He can help by placing his hands on the chair arms and helping to lower himself into the chair, if possible. Check your feet position. If you are pivoting correctly, yours and your loved one's feet will be parallel.

Moving Into the Car

Your loved one's situation may make it difficult for you to take him places in the car. It can take extra time and effort to help him in and out of the car, to put a wheelchair or other assistive device in the car, or to deal with your loved one's behaviors such as agitation or confusion. Try not to let these things stop you from taking your loved one places. Being homebound can lead to frustration and isolation.

To make transportation more enjoyable and safer, follow these tips from Easter Seals:

- Give yourself and your loved one extra time to get in and out of the car. The slower you go, the faster things get done.
- When you are going to a new place with your loved one for the first time, call ahead and find out which entrance to use. This way you can avoid getting in and out of the car multiple times.
- Prepare to be comfortable. Plan to have the things you need such as relaxing music, sunglasses, food and water, and some photos to calm him. Be prepared for temperature changes. Keep the vehicle clutter-free, and try to reduce glare on bright days.
- Ask your loved one to use the bathroom before you leave.

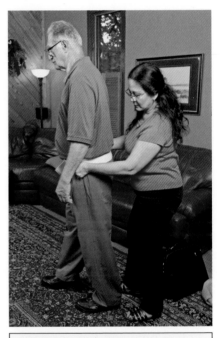

Using a gait belt will give you something to grip while helping your loved one walk.

- When communicating with your loved one, speak clearly in a calm and respectful tone. Give brief, clear directions (step-by-step if necessary) to avoid confusion. Make eye contact when possible.

- Show or demonstrate to your loved one what you would like him to do.
- Choose pleasant topics of conversation in the car and avoid arguing during your outing.

Moving from Wheelchair to Car

- Have the person wear a gait belt, if one is available.
- Open the car door.
- Stand with your back to the inside of the car door and pull the wheelchair toward you — between the car door and seat. Set the brakes of the wheelchair.
- Talk your loved one through the transfer process step-by-step so he can assist if possible.
- Hold on to the gait belt and help him to a standing position — use your legs for strength as you pull.
- Have your loved one lean forward, toward you, and put his arms around your shoulders (not your neck), if possible.
- Carefully pivot yourself and your loved one so his backside is toward the inside of the car.
- Help him sit on the seat with his legs still out of the car — be careful that he bends at the waist so his head clears the door frame and he sits down squarely on the car seat.
- Once he is sitting, give him a moment to gain his balance. Help move his legs into the car (a swivel cushion is helpful for this).
- Assist with the seat belt and close the door before going to the driver's seat.

Make certain your loved one's seat belt is securely fastened while in transit and that he does not unfasten it until the vehicle comes to a complete stop. Provide assistance when he enters or exits the vehicle, but do not make him feel rushed. Give your loved one extra time to do what is needed.

Learn more at www.EasterSeals.org. Click on *Site Map*, scroll down to *Mobility* then click on

◎ If Your Loved One Begins to Fall

1. If possible, help stabilize him or lower him to the ground. To maintain proper body mechanics, keep your feet apart, back straight and knees slightly bent. Place your forward, flexed leg or hip against your loved one's back, thigh or buttocks.

2. Put your arms around his waist or underarms, keep him close to your body, bend your knees and lower him slowly to the floor by sliding him down your leg.

3. Check to see if he is injured. Check for pain or bleeding.

4. Call the health-care provider after your loved one falls. If you suspect head, neck or back injury, **CALL 9-1-1**.

5. If he is not injured, and if possible, help him up into a chair or into bed.

Transportation Solutions for Caregivers in the left hand column.

Helping Your Loved One Walk

Your loved one may use a walker, a cane or crutches. He may have trouble walking after spending a lot of time in bed. If your loved one is unsteady, encourage him to practice standing by balancing between two sturdy supports, such as the backs of heavy chairs.

When your loved one is stronger and more confident, the next step is walking without holding on to the chairs. At first, walk with your loved one. If you place a gait belt around his waist there will be something for you to grip. Grip the belt from behind so you will not be in the way as he walks forward. Your loved one may tend to watch his feet or the floor when walking. Encourage him to have good posture and to stand up straight

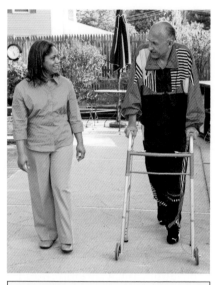

Remind your loved one to walk as normally as possible while using the walker for stability.

and hold his head high. If your loved one is weak or afraid of falling, walk with your hands on his waist from behind or around his waist from the side.

Using a Walker

1. Put the walker directly in front of your loved one.
2. Help him to stand. Do not let him pull on the walker to

stand up as it can fall.

3. Ask him to put his hands on the walker's handgrips. The height of the walker should be at about the same height as his hipbone.

4. Ask him to flex his elbows slightly.

5. Have your loved one lift or roll the walker about 6 inches forward and then step into it.

Remind him to use the walker to support himself as he stands on one leg and moves his other leg forward. He should use his arms to hold himself up if his legs are weak.

If the walker has no wheels and your loved one has trouble lifting it, cut a hole in four tennis balls and attach them to the feet of the walker. This will make sliding it easier.

Remind your loved one to look ahead and walk as normally as possible while using the walker for stability.

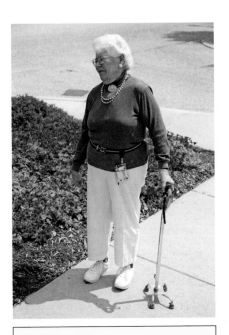

Put the cane near your loved one's stronger side.

Using a Cane

1. Use a four-pronged cane for better stability. Put the cane near your loved one's stronger hand and have him put his hand on the handle. Make sure the top of the cane is even with his hipbone and the bottom is 6 inches from his foot.

2. Ask him to flex his elbow slightly.
3. Have your loved one support himself as he stands on his stronger side and moves his weaker leg forward.
4. Walk on your loved one's weaker side or behind him to assist if necessary.
5. Encourage him to practice walking normally — always looking ahead — while using the cane.

Walking Without an Assistive Device

1. Stand at your loved one's side where you can provide the most support; usually this is the strong side.
2. Encourage him to walk normally and to look ahead.
3. Gradually increase the distance he walks to help him build confidence and endurance.

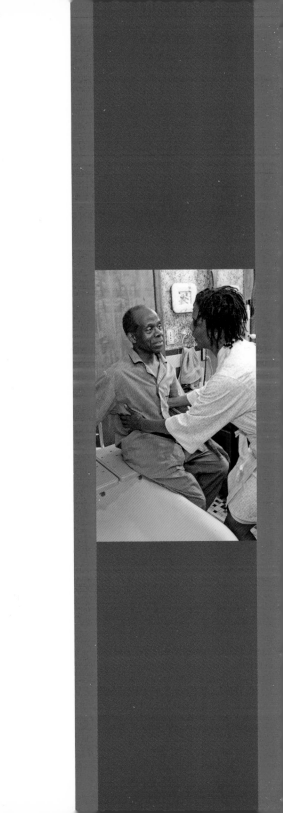

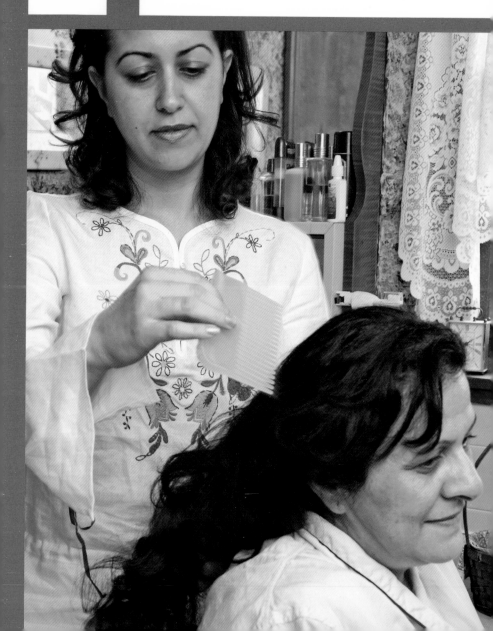

4

Personal Care

"The one thing I learned pretty quickly when helping Mom with personal care is to not treat her like a child," says Diane, whose mother suffers from Alzheimer's disease. "Some days she can dress, wash and brush her own teeth and I just stand by to assist and encourage her. Other times she lets me help. But sometimes she won't do it at all, so I just wait a little while and try again."

Grooming

A clean, well-groomed appearance can improve your loved one's sense of well-being and make her feel better about herself. Become her personal care partner by encouraging her to do what she can and helping with tasks she finds difficult.

If your loved one is able, you might want to consider trips to a local hair salon or barbershop. Getting up and out of the house can be refreshing for your loved one and may help improve her mood and outlook.

Assisting with your loved one's personal needs, such as dressing, eating, bathing and going to the bathroom, can be an enjoyable time together once you get over any initial awkwardness.

Deciding what to wear, when to get up and how to style her hair will help your loved one maintain a positive self-image and sense of independence.

Personal care tasks will be easier if you set aside time in your daily routine to make sure your loved one is clean, safe and comfortable. A representative schedule is shown on the opposite page.

Brushing and Combing Hair
Ask your loved one how she would like her hair styled each day. Encourage her to look in the mirror as you groom her hair. Some medications and medical treatments cause hair to become brittle or to fall out, so always brush hair gently. Start at the ends and work gradually toward the scalp in small sections.

Your loved one may like to use oils, creams or lotions that make the hair easier to comb and that moisturize the scalp. These are usually applied after shampooing and massaged into the scalp and hair.

If your loved one's hair is tangled, use a comb with widely spaced, blunt teeth and work slowly. For extremely tangled

Personal Care Schedule

Time of Day	Personal Care Needs
Morning	Go to the bathroom
	Wash face and hands, comb hair
	Bathe
	Brush teeth, or clean dentures
	Get dressed
During the day	Take care of any personal needs that arise before and after mealtimes, exercise and giving medications.
	Offer help with toileting as quickly as possible whenever your loved one feels an urge to use the bathroom.
Evening	Undress and change into nightclothes
	Go to the bathroom
	Wash face and hands
	Brush and floss teeth, or clean dentures
	Make sure bed linens are smooth, dry and wrinkle-free
	Offer fresh drinking water
	Take care of any other personal needs

hair, wet the hair first and apply conditioner before combing. Rinse after you have removed the tangles. Coarse hair also may be easier to comb while it is wet.

Be sure to report any unusual conditions, such as sores on the scalp, to the health-care provider.

Shaving

Help your loved one into a sitting position and put a towel over his chest.

Before you begin, inspect his skin for moles, birthmarks or sores. Shave carefully around these areas. Keep in mind that certain medical disorders and some medications can cause

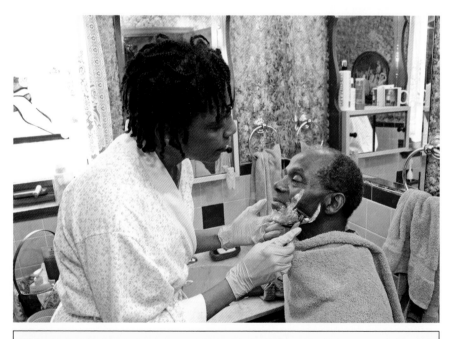

Take care to avoid cutting yourself or your loved one when handling a razor blade.

excessive bleeding if a person is cut.

With the fingers of one hand, hold the skin tight in the area you are shaving and work downward toward your loved one's neck under his chin. Shave only in the direction hair grows – downwards.

If your loved one has a curly beard, he may prefer to use depilatory cream or powder to remove facial hair instead of shaving.

Encourage him to use aftershave lotion because the alcohol acts as an antiseptic.

Safety Razor. Safety razors may hold replaceable blades or be disposable. Take care to avoid cutting yourself or your loved one when handling a razor blade.

- Soften the beard first by placing a warm washcloth on the lower half of his face for 3 to 5 minutes. Shaving cream also softens the beard and helps the razor glide over the skin.
- Use short strokes around your loved one's chin and lips and rinse the razor often to remove hair.
- When finished, remove any remaining shaving cream with a wet washcloth and help him pat dry with a towel.
- Place the razor end down in a container, but don't recap it.

Electric Shaver. Your loved one may prefer to use an electric shaver. Use an electric razor instead of a safety razor if your loved one has a blood-clotting disorder or if he takes medication that affects how fast the blood clots.

However, do not use an electric shaver on someone using oxygen therapy as it could spark a fire.

For safety, first check the condition of the shaver to make sure that the screen has no holes and the cord isn't frayed. To prevent electrocution, keep electric shavers away from water.

Use the shaver as the manufacturer suggests, usually in a circular motion. Keep the shaver in good working order; take it apart and clean it when finished. Always unplug electrical appliances before cleaning.

Hands and Fingernails

Your loved one may need help with handwashing. Both of you should wash your hands often each day, especially before eating and after going to the bathroom.

Keep fingernails trimmed and smooth to help prevent injury to the skin. Use caution to avoid cutting the skin, espe-

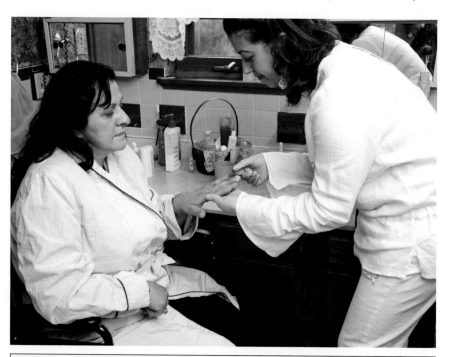

Keep fingernails trimmed and smooth to help prevent injury.

cially when trimming the nails of a person who has diabetes, poor circulation, paralysis, decreased sensation in the hand or is taking blood-thinning medications.

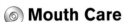

Mouth Care

Mouth care is important for your loved one's health and comfort. Be gentle and allow enough time. Also, be sure to observe any changes in your loved one's mouth and report anything unusual to the health-care provider.

- Use a toothbrush with soft bristles and replace it every 3 to 6 months, or as soon as it shows wear.
- Mix mouthwash with water to help protect your loved one's gums.
- To control the amount of saliva produced, brush the upper teeth first, then the lower teeth.

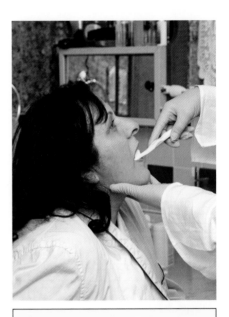

Use a toothbrush with soft bristles and replace it every 3 to 6 months.

Denture Care

Your loved one may wear complete (full-mouth) dentures or partial dentures. Wearing dentures prevents the gums from shrinking and maintains the mouth's natural shape. It also improves a person's speech, makes eating easier and improves a person's self-

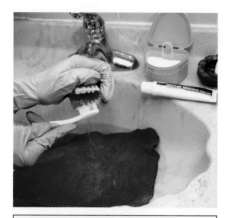

When cleaning dentures, handle carefully.

image. Provide mouth care after dentures are removed.

Remind your loved one to remove her dentures for at least 8 hours each day to rest her gums (usually at bedtime).

Handle dentures carefully so they do not chip or break.

Dressing

Even though it takes some time and effort on your part, it is important to your loved one's self-esteem to dress in regular clothes every day. Getting dressed helps your loved one maintain her sense of identity. Allow her to decide what outfit to wear. Making choices is a sign of independence. If she has difficulty making decisions, help her decide by giving her two outfits from which to choose.

When helping your loved one select clothing, consider her likes and dislikes, what is easiest to put on and take off, weather conditions, temperature and planned activities.

How to Help

When helping with dressing, prevent your loved one from falling by having her sit down on a chair or the side of a bed. If she is not stable sitting up, help her lie down in bed and cover her with a sheet or towel for warmth and privacy.

As you help your loved one get dressed and undressed, observe her skin for any redness, skin irritation or abnormalities and report these to the health-care provider.

Undressing. When undressing, start removing his clothes at his chest and work your way down. To provide privacy for a woman, put a sheet or towel over her shoulders and upper body before completely removing her top.

If the top must come off over her head, pull it off her strongest arm first. She can use the other arm to hold the blanket or towel over herself.

To remove pants from someone who is lying down, ask her

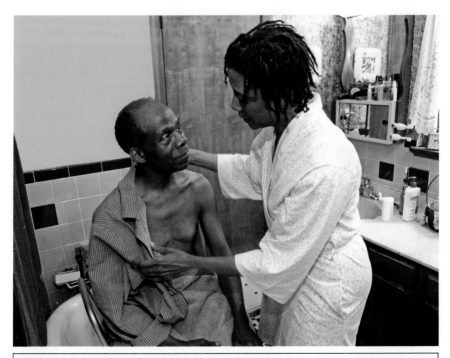

When undressing your loved one, prevent him from falling by having him sit down on a chair or on the side of a bed.

to raise her hips so you can reach under the sheet to help slip the pants down over the hips. If she cannot raise her hips, turn her on her side and pull the pants down over her buttocks and hip on that side. Repeat the process on the other side.

Dressing. When dressing, begin with her feet and work your way up.

Help her put on socks first, then help her put on underwear and pants part way. Put on her shoes and help her stand so you can pull up the underwear and pants.

If she is lying down, ask her to raise her hips, if possible, so you can pull up her underwear and pants.

If she has a weak or paralyzed side, dress that side first so clothes are loose when being pulled over the stiff or sore side.

When helping a woman put on her bra, hook it in front and

turn it around. Then help guide her arms into the straps.

Bathing, Showering and Shampooing

Your loved one's health and physical capabilities will help determine whether she bathes and shampoos in the bed, the shower or the tub. Ask her what she prefers and then consider how you can assist.

Make sure showers and tubs have nonskid mats and surfaces and that shower chairs and grab bars are fastened tightly to the wall.

Check the water temperature with a bath thermometer or by touching the inside of your wrist to the water. Water temperature should be lower than 105° F.

Make sure the room is warm and that there are no drafts.

Inspect your loved one's skin for injuries, changes in condition and color (reddened areas or sores).

When finished with bathing, make sure all soap and shampoo is thoroughly rinsed, and help her out of the tub or shower, making sure she steps onto a nonskid surface.

After helping her towel off, apply lotion if she likes. But if you apply lotion to her feet, immediately have her put on socks or slippers so she does not slip on the floor.

Cleaning the Genital Area
Practice proper infection control measures by wearing disposable gloves when washing your loved one's genitals and open

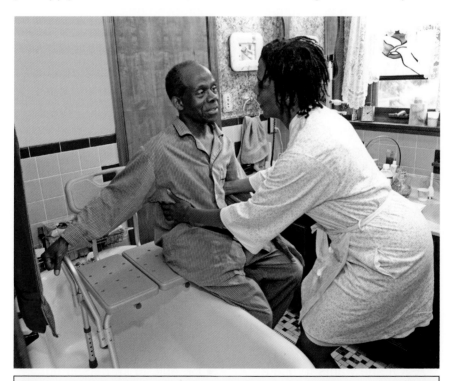

When tub bathing your loved one, help him into the tub or tub chair.

wound areas. Or, ask if she wants to do this task herself.

Whether assisting a man or a woman, always wash the genitals from front to back (towards the anus). Cleaning in this direction avoids contaminating the urethral opening with bacteria from the anal area.

For both men and women, use a different part of the washcloth for each stroke to prevent the spread of germs.

Showering

Many people enjoy bathing and shampooing in the shower. If your loved one is steady on her feet, she may be able to stand in the shower. Beware of slips and falls. She may need a shower chair or shower seat. Before helping your loved one shower, determine whether you need special safety equipment. If using a shower chair, lock the brakes or place the chair against the shower wall.

Ask if she wants to use a shower cap, give her soap and encourage her to wash as much as possible. If she wants to wash her own hair, stand by to provide help if needed.

Tub Bathing

Most problems and falls occur when getting out of the tub. To determine if it is safe for your loved one to use the bathtub, she should:

- Be predictable. This means her behavior would not be unexpected and she does not suffer from an illness, such as dementia, that would affect her behavior.
- Be able to reliably bear all or most of her own weight when standing.
- Be able to stand on one foot and lift the other foot over the edge of the tub with minimal assistance.
- Be able to lower her body onto the tub seat or into the tub.
- Be able to lift herself out of the tub.

Fill the tub halfway with warm water. Shut off the hot water first to prevent hot water in the faucet from dripping onto your loved one's skin.

Help your loved one into the tub or tub chair and offer a towel to cover her shoulders if she seemes chilled. Encourage her to wash herself as much as possible.

Bed Bathing

If your loved one is unable to get out of bed, he will need a bed bath. When a full bath is not needed, you may want to wash only his face, hands, armpits, genital area, back and buttocks. Encourage your loved one to do as much as he can.

If your loved one is able, you may suggest that he wash

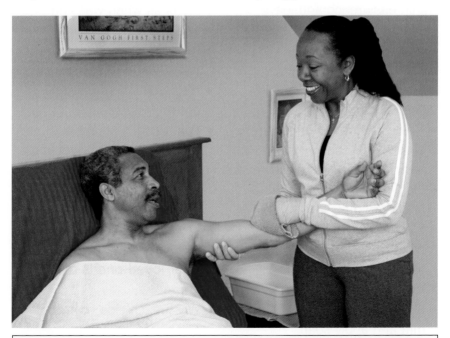

If your loved one is unable to get out of bed, he will need a bed bath.

his own genitals. After making sure he is safe, hand him the washcloth and provide privacy.

Bathing the Genital Area.
Wash the genital area last. Place a towel under the buttocks to protect the bed. If your loved one can do this himself, place the washcloth, soap, towel and water basin within easy reach and leave him alone for privacy if it is safe to do so.

   If your loved one cannot wash his or her own genitals, follow these specific procedures:

- Cover your loved one from stomach to chest with a flannel sheet or large towel.
- Help him bend his knees and spread his legs.
- Elevate his hips by placing either a bedpan or a folded towel under the buttocks.
- Put on disposable gloves.
- Make the washcloth into a mitt and apply soap.
- Always wash and dry the genital area from front to back to avoid bringing germs forward from the rectal area.
- Wash the pubic hair on the pelvic region.
- Rinse the soap out of the washcloth. Rinse the genital area by following the same steps as when washing.
- Dry the genital area with a clean towel, using the same steps as when washing and rinsing.
- Remove the bedpan or folded towel.
- Help your loved one roll onto his side.
- Wash and rinse the anal area. Move in the direction away from the genital area. Use a different area of the washcloth for each stroke.
- Dry the anal area thoroughly.

If your loved one is a woman:
- Wash each side of her vagina in one gentle, even stroke, then wash gently

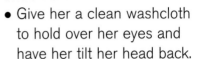

down the middle using a different area of the washcloth for each stroke.

- If the woman in your care is menstruating, put a clean menstrual pad in place after washing and voiding.

If your loved one is a man:

- Wash the tip of his penis with a soapy washcloth. Always wash from the opening outward in a circular motion.
- Rinse the soap from the washcloth. Rinse and pat dry the penis tip using the same steps as when washing.
- Wash, rinse and pat dry the shaft of the penis. If the man in your care is not circumcised, gently push back the foreskin and clean around any loose skin. Gently pat the area dry and move the foreskin back over the end of the penis.
- Wash, rinse and pat dry his scrotum and surrounding area thoroughly.

Shampooing

If shampooing your loved one's hair:

- Give her a clean washcloth to hold over her eyes and have her tilt her head back.
- Using a plastic pitcher, pour water over her head to wet the hair thoroughly.
- Shampoo and rinse her hair. Use conditioner, if needed.
- Dry her hair and wrap her head with the towel.

Assisting with Toileting

It's normal for you or your loved one to feel shy about helping and needing help with a very personal function. Be sensitive to those feelings.

When assisting with toileting, provide privacy by closing the door, but let her know that you will stay nearby to help if needed.

Give your loved one as much time as necessary but check on her regularly so you do not leave her stranded on the bed-

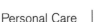

pan or alone in the bathroom too long. Encourage her to remain on the toilet for a few minutes to make sure the bladder is empty.

If you are caring for a loved one who is too ill to get out of bed, you will have to help her use a bedpan for urinating and bowel movements.

Using a Urinal

The urinal is a bottle-shaped container that men use. If necessary, help your loved one with the urinal by placing it between his legs and, while wearing disposable gloves, gently put his penis into the opening.

Leave a call bell or other signal within easy reach, and if it is safe to do so, leave the room to give him privacy.

After use, remove the urinal promptly, cover it and take it to the bathroom. Help your loved one wash his hands.

After checking the urine for anything unusual, empty the urinal into the toilet and clean it with cool soapy water, then rinse. Keep the urinal out of sight when not in use.

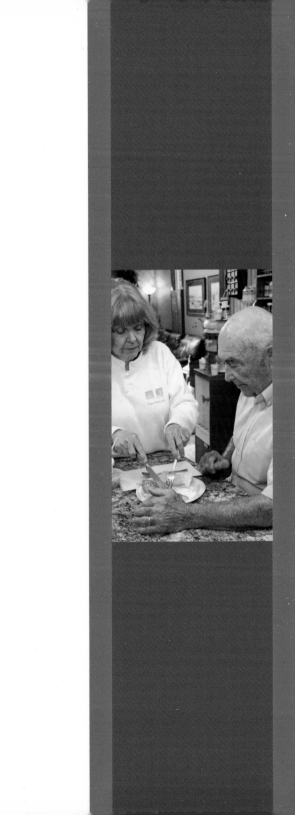

5

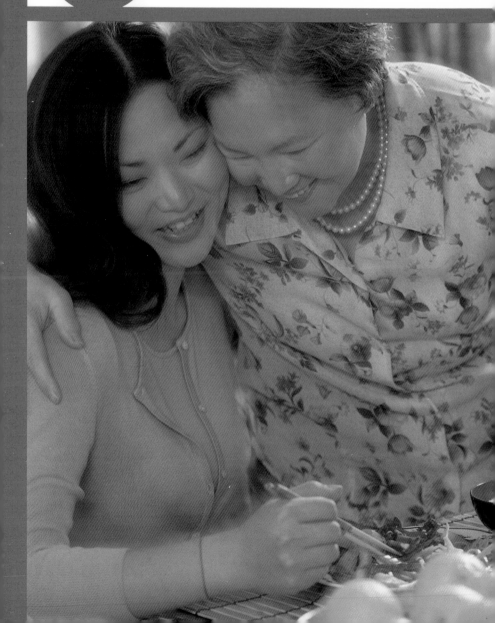

Healthy Eating

"One of the positive things about having Mom move in with us was family dinners," recalls Debbie, whose mother had Parkinson's disease. "Mom really wanted the family to eat dinner together with the TV off. I think we eat better when we eat together."

tips

Make Mealtime Enjoyable

Making mealtime as pleasant as possible will help encourage your loved one to eat better. Here are some tips:

☐ Let your loved one help plan each day's meals. Ask what foods he does and doesn't like.

☐ Keep the atmosphere as cheerful as possi- ble and provide enough lighting.

☐ Keep the room neat, clean and free of odors.

☐ Attractive meals are more appetizing. Use colorful plates and napkins. Include something special on the tray such as a flower or favorite magazine.

Nutrition Is Important

Follow good nutrition and healthful eating habits for your- self, your family and the loved one in your care. Make grains, fruits and vegetables a regular part of your meals. Limit fat, sugars, salt and alcohol. For the loved one in your care, follow the health-care provider and dietitian's recommendations and make mealtime enjoyable for your whole family.

Malnutrition can be a serious problem for people who are ill or elderly because they may not be hungry or they may have difficulty eating. But proper nutrition is important because it can help sick or injured people feel better and recover faster.

For example, if your loved one has diabetes, he may need to eat less carbohydrates as well as fewer total calories each day. Or, if your loved one is recovering from a burn or open sore, eating more protein and increasing total calories may promote healing. A less active person may need fewer total calories than someone who expends more energy. If your loved one eats only small servings, he may need to eat a healthy snack or another small meal between meals.

Select a variety of foods including grains, vegetables, fruit, meat, beans, milk, and limited amounts of fats, oils, and sweets. For guidance on how to best meet your loved one's special nutritional needs, ask his health-care provider or dietitian.

Preparing for a Meal

Set up a schedule for mealtime and stick to it so your loved one doesn't get upset by frequent changes. However, if he is not hungry at mealtime and wants to eat later, be flexible.

Your loved one may feel better prepared to enjoy meals after attending to personal care. Before breakfast, allow

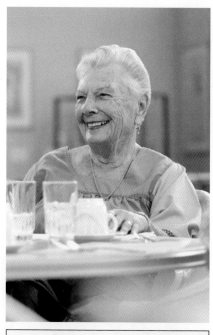

Making mealtime pleasant will help encourage your loved one to eat better.

time for washing, grooming, dressing and dental or denture care, and provide help if necessary. Before other meals, encourage him to go to the bathroom and wash his hands before eating.

Always use clean utensils

and napkins and protect your loved one's clothing with a napkin or towel.

Have your loved one sit in a comfortable, upright position. Having his head up and the hips at a 90-degree angle will make it easier for him to chew, swallow and manage eating utensils.

Serve meals promptly to make sure hot food stays hot and cold food stays cold.

Helping Your Loved One Eat

Observe your loved one during mealtime to find out what kind of help he needs. This will probably depend on the food being served and how tired he is. If you give more help than

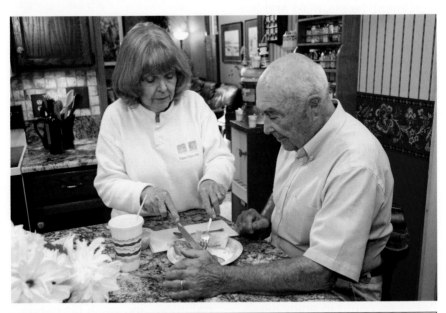

Make sure your loved one is comfortable and positioned correctly for eating, using a chair that pulls close to the table.

needed you may make your loved one feel helpless, so encourage him to do as much as possible on his own.

You may find that a certain task, such as cutting meat, is more difficult for him to manage than eating a sandwich. If this is the case, try to serve finger foods, or foods prepared in bite-size pieces more often.

Make sure your loved one is comfortable and positioned correctly for eating. If possible, use a dining room or kitchen chair that pulls close to the table. Make sure his feet are flat on the floor, and have him rest his elbows or forearms on the table for support if needed. Place a towel or napkin over his chest to protect his clothing.

Sometimes people leave part of a meal uneaten because they are too tired to finish. If your loved one appears tired, offer to help him eat more and offer a snack later in the day.

To help make eating easier, your loved one's health-care provider may recommend certain assistive devices, such as special cups, plates, bowls, eating utensils and straws. These are available from medical supply companies.

Make sure food and dishes are not too hot. Wait until food stops steaming or the plate has cooled a little before serving a meal. Test the temperature of hot liquids by placing several drops on your wrist. If the liquid feels too hot, allow it to cool slightly before serving it. Offer liquids only when your loved one has no food in his mouth.

Giving Liquids by Straw

To offer a liquid by straw, place the straw in your loved one's mouth. He can suck and swallow the liquid as desired. If your loved one sucks too much liquid, you may have to pinch off the straw and pull it away so he can swallow.

Make sure the liquids are

never hot. Serving liquid at the correct temperature is especially important if your loved one drinks hot liquid through a straw because the liquid bypasses the lips as the straw delivers liquid far back in the mouth, where it could cause serious burns to the mouth and throat if it is too hot.

If your loved one has trouble swallowing, he may have problems using a straw. Talk with the health-care provider about your concerns.

Giving Liquids by Cup

To offer fluids by cup to a loved one who is not sitting up, raise and support his head with one hand and hold the cup with your other hand while he drinks. Remove the cup often to let him swallow. Adult (or child) spill-proof cups can make it easier for your loved one to drink. These cups are available in many sizes, with or without straws.

Help with Feeding

Offer a liquid first to moisten the mouth and make it easier to swallow. Then fill a spoon no more than two-thirds full and touch the spoon to his bottom lip so that he opens his mouth. Touch the spoon to the tongue. Touching the lips and tongue lets your loved one know where the spoon is in his mouth.

Feed him slowly, and allow time between bites for him to chew and swallow. Name each food as you offer it. Wipe his mouth with a napkin, as needed.

Offer liquids after several swallows of solid food, making sure the liquids are not too hot. End the meal with water to rinse the mouth.

When he is finished eating, remove the dishes and clean up the table. Help him wash his hands and brush his teeth or rinse his mouth.

Trouble Seeing

If he has trouble seeing, you may be able to help him eat independently, without having to feed him. Talking about the food during the meal may help your loved one visualize it and feed himself. Describe the foods on the table and their locations as if the plate were the face of a clock. For example, say, "The green beans are at 8 o'clock. The potatoes are at 4 o'clock." Also describe the location of the eating utensils. Cut up the meat or anything else that needs cutting and open any containers.

Check to see whether your loved one has missed any of the food on his plate and, if so, offer assistance.

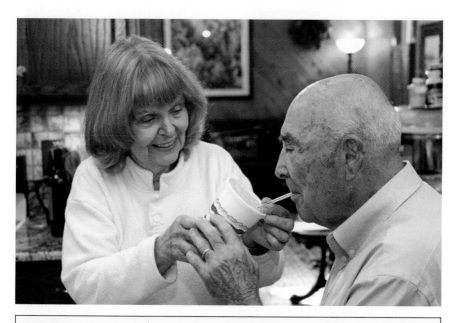

If your loved one sucks too much liquid, you may have to pinch off the straw and pull it away so he can swallow.

Trouble Swallowing

If your loved one has trouble swallowing or often chokes, gags or coughs during eating, be sure to discuss this with his health-care provider and remain with him while he is eating.

If a stroke left your loved one with speech difficulties, he may also have trouble swallowing food. The health-care provider and speech therapist will order an appropriate diet. Generally, soft foods are easier to swallow than liquids, which run down the throat.

If he has swallowing difficulties, place food toward the back of the mouth, on the unaffected side, because if he cannot feel food on the paralyzed side it may accumulate in his cheek.

Check your loved one's mouth during and after the meal. Food that remains in the mouth could cause choking.

If your loved one is unable to safely swallow food other than purees, or if his swallow is extremely slow, you may need to find ways to increase the calories he consumes. Increase calories in purees by adding extra butter, margarine, mayonnaise, syrups, gravies or sauces in meals.

Encourage him to tilt his chin down as he swallows. When you help feed your loved one, have him sit up. Keep his head elevated during meals and for at least 30 minutes afterward. Encourage him to chew slowly and thoroughly. Allow enough time for eating. Hurrying could increase the likelihood of choking.

Eliminate distractions, such as television or too many visitors, so that he can concentrate on eating. Observe your loved one as he eats to watch for choking, and know how to respond.

Appetite Matters

Chronically ill people often lose

◎ How to Respond to Choking

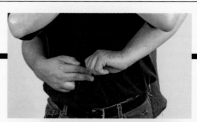

The Red Cross strongly recommends that you take a first aid/CPR/AED course to learn how to respond to choking. Here's what to do:

Check the scene and the person.

- Send someone to **CALL 9-1-1** or the local emergency number and get permission to provide care.
- If coughing, encourage the person to continue to cough.

If an adult is unable to cough, speak or breathe (choking).

- Lean the person forward and give 5 back blows between the shoulder blades with the heel of your hand.
- Give 5 quick, upward abdominal thrusts.
  - Place thumbside of fist against middle of

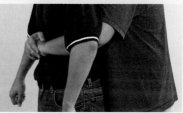

abdomen just above the navel.
- Grab fist with the other hand.

Repeat back blows and abdominal thrusts until:

- Object is forced out and person breathes or coughs forcefully on his or her own.
- Person becomes unconscious.
- If the person becomes unconscious **CALL 9-1-1** or the local emergency number, if you, or someone else, has not already done so.

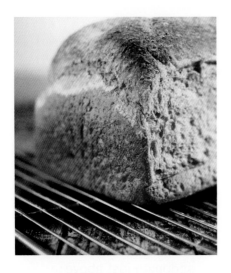

the smell of bread in the oven may make one person hungry, but make another feel sick. Smell also affects taste; a person who can't smell food, can't taste much either. That's one reason why somone who is congested may not feel hungry.

It usually takes a few days for a poor appetite to improve. Be patient. If your loved one isn't hungry, offer food again later.

their appetite, which can lead to malnutrition. Many things can affect your loved one's appetite. For example, he may not feel hungry if he is ill or nauseated. Some medications could also cause him to lose his appetite or feel extra hungry. Appetite can also be suppressed by emotions such as happiness, excitement, loneliness or grief.

You should also be aware that the smell of food can have an unpredictable effect on a person's appetite. For example,

Fluids Are Important

To maintain good health, a person must consume enough fluid to replace the fluid lost each day. For most people that's about 6 to 8 cups. The fluid can be in liquid form, such as water, coffee, juice, milk, soup and tea, or in solid form, such as ice cream, sherbet or gelatin.

Some illnesses or conditions make it more important to be aware of how much fluid your loved one drinks and how much passes through his body. For example, if he perspires heavily (as with a fever), vomits (as with a stomach virus) or has diarrhea, he must drink liquids to replace lost fluids quickly.

Even when he is well, your loved one's fluid balance may be off simply because he doesn't drink enough. Perhaps he is afraid he won't get to the bathroom in time. Or he may be sick or have a disability — such as arthritis — that makes it difficult to get up to get a drink or to hold a glass. Your loved one may be afraid that he might spill the liquid. Or he may simply forget to drink fluids.

Whatever its cause, dehydration is a serious condition. If your loved one is losing a lot of fluid or is dehydrated, notify the health-care provider immediately. Symptoms of dehydration include: confusion; nausea; low blood pressure; rapid pulse rate; dry mouth; weakness; constipation; drowsiness; very dry skin or chapped lips; decreased urination or scanty, dark-colored

tips

To Encourage Hydration

☐ Offer drinks your loved one likes, at the preferred temperature, several times throughout the day.

☐ Do not limit beverages in hope of having fewer trips to the bathroom.

☐ Encourage your loved one to drink plenty of fluids with meals.

☐ Provide him with a pitcher of clean, fresh water and a clean drinking glass or cup within easy reach.

☐ Encourage him to drink throughout the day.

☐ Refill the glass if he cannot do it.

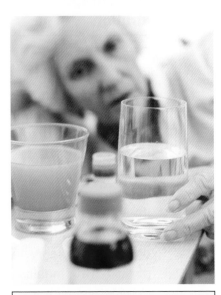

When your loved one has diarrhea, she should drink plenty of fluids.

urine; elevated temperature; decreased sweat in armpits and groin; soft eyeballs; and skin that stays in a tent shape when you gently pinch it.

Diarrhea

With diarrhea, food passes quickly through the bowel — more than 8 loose stools in 24 hours — resulting in dehydra-tion. Diarrhea may have several causes, including cancer treatment, infection, food sensitivities, gastrointestinal problems and emotional upset. If your loved one has diarrhea that lasts more than 2 days, notify his health-care provider. Ways to cope with diarrhea include:

- Drink plenty of fluids to replenish what is lost.
- Eat small meals throughout the day instead of three larger meals.
- Eat plenty of foods containing salt and potassium (such as beef broth for sodium; bananas and potatoes for potassium).
- Try a soft diet.
- Your loved one may also need to avoid high-fat, greasy foods, such as steak and french fries, as well as milk products. The lactose in milk products may worsen diarrhea. If the diarrhea does not go away in a couple of days, try clear liquids for 24 hours and contact the health-care

provider.

Nausea and Vomiting

Nausea and vomiting may be caused by cancer treatments, medication side effects, food odors, gas in the stomach or bowel or motion sickness.

If vomiting is severe or lasts more than a couple of days, notify your loved one's health-care provider. Here are some tips to control vomiting:

- Do not give your loved one anything to eat until the vomiting is under control.
- Give small amounts of clear liquids.
- When your loved one is able to keep down clear liquids, try a thicker liquid or soft diet.
- During bouts of nausea, offer your loved one some of these foods: dry toast, crackers, sherbet, angel food cake, cooked cereal, boiled potato, rice or noodles, skinned baked chicken and carbonated beverages.
- Do not give your loved one high-fat, greasy foods or foods that are too spicy or have strong odors.
- Give your loved one small amounts of foods throughout the day and fluids between meals.
- Help your loved one gradually work up to his normal healthy diet.

Monitoring Intake and Output

The health-care provider may want to know how much food and fluids your loved one is taking in each day. He or she may also ask you to keep a record of bowel movements, urine and/or vomit as well.

If so, keep a record of foods served, the time and the amount eaten. Each time he finishes drinking a container of liquid, record the amount in a notebook. You may also want to include comments about your loved one's appetite and mood at mealtime.

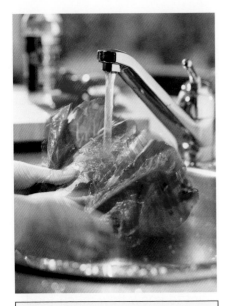

Rinse raw fruits and vegetables with running water before eating.

Keep Food Safe to Eat

Eating foods that contain harmful bacteria, viruses or toxins can cause foodborne illness. Even a few bites of an unsafe food may make you or your loved one sick. Children, the elderly and people with weakened immune systems or chronic illnesses are at a high risk of foodborne illness.

Wash Hands and Surfaces Often

- Wash your hands vigorously for at least 15 seconds before handling food or utensils.
- Wash your hands after handling food, especially after handling raw meat, poultry, fish or eggs.
- After preparing foods, wash the utensils and surfaces you used with hot, soapy water.
- Rinse raw fruits and vegetables with running water before eating. Use a vegetable brush to remove any dirt.

Store Food Safely

- Separate raw, cooked and ready-to-eat foods while shopping, preparing and storing.
- Keep raw meat, poultry,

eggs and fish away from other foods, surfaces, utensils and dishes to prevent contamination.

- Store raw meat, poultry and fish in containers on the lower shelves of the refrigerator so that the juices don't drip onto other foods.
- Keep a thermometer in the refrigerator and freezer to ensure that foods are being stored at the right temperature. Your refrigerator should be under 40° F. The freezer should be less than 0° F.
- If your refrigerator power goes off, discard foods that might have been kept at room temperature for 2 hours or more.
- Do not thaw foods in a sink stopped up with water.
- Never thaw meat, poultry, fish or shellfish at room temperature.

Cook Safely

Proper cooking makes most uncooked foods safe, but uncooked or undercooked foods can be unsafe to eat.

The best way to tell if meat, poultry or egg dishes are cooked to a safe temperature is to use a food thermometer.

- Reheat sauces, soups and gravies to a boil.
- Reheat leftovers thoroughly to at least 165° F.
- Cook eggs until whites and yolks are firm.
- Don't eat raw or partially cooked eggs or foods containing raw eggs.
- Cook fish and shellfish until they are opaque; fish should flake easily with a fork.
- Cook poultry to 180° F internal temperature.

Refrigerate Foods That Can Spoil Quickly

- When shopping for food, select perishable items (foods that can spoil) last, and take

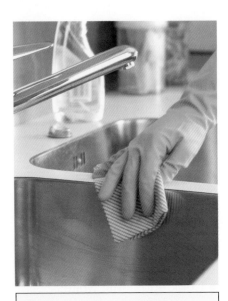

To prevent germs from spreading, clean up with warm, soapy water.

them home right away.

- Refrigerate or freeze meat, poultry, eggs, fish, shellfish and ready-to-eat foods promptly.
- Refrigerate food within 2 hours of purchasing or preparation and within 1 hour if the air temperature is above 90° F.
- Freeze leftovers or use

refrigerated leftovers within 3 to 4 days.

- Freeze fresh meat, poultry, fish and shellfish that will not be used in a few days.
- Thaw frozen meat, poultry, fish and shellfish in the refrigerator, in the microwave as part of the cooking process or under cold running water that covers the surface of the meat.
- Cook foods immediately after thawing.
- Follow safety instructions on food labels, such as "Keep refrigerated."

Serve Foods Safely

- Keep hot foods hot (140° F or above) and cold foods cold (41° F or below).
- Use separate cutting boards for meats, vegetables and ready-to-eat foods to prevent contamination.
- Never leave meat, luncheon meat, dairy products, poultry, eggs, fish or shellfish out at

room temperature for more than 2 hours.

- To prevent the spread of germs, do not sip, blow on or touch your loved one's food to check the temperature.

Clean Up

After mealtime, dispose of left-over food as soon as possible. Dispose of liquids in the sink or flush them down the toilet. Put leftover soft and solid foods in a garbage disposal or place them in a plastic bag before putting them in the trashcan to keep pests away.

To prevent germs from spreading, use your diswasher or wash all dishes and utensils with warm, soapy water and rinse them with hot water. Allow the dishes and utensils to drain and dry on a rack instead of drying them with a dish towel.

Dietary Concerns

Be sure to tell the health-care provider exactly what dietary supplements, including vita-mins, fiber, minerals, herbs and food supplements, your loved one is taking. In most instances, the supplements should not replace all solid foods.

Food Allergies and Sensitivities

Your loved one may be allergic or sensitive to some foods such as eggs, milk, wheat or peanuts. Other common allergies include shellfish and fish, tree nuts and soy. Food allergy or sensitivity may cause: diarrhea; red, itchy skin; nausea and/or stomach pain; vomiting; wheezing or coughing; hives; shortness of breath; sneezing and watery eyes; swelling of the throat, face, mouth or lips; severe gas; muscle cramps; or dizziness.

A person with severe food allergies can have an allergic reaction from simply touching or smelling the food. The reaction typically occurs within a few minutes to 1 hour after

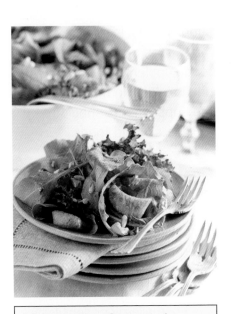

Make grains, fruits and vegetables a regular part of your meals.

Special Diets

If the health-care provider orders a special diet for your loved one, ask questions and get detailed information from him or her on what foods your loved one should eat. Ask for a referral to a dietition to advise you on how to adhere to the diet. Then make sure your loved one gets only the food permitted in that diet. Eating food that is not recommended can cause health problems.

High-protein diet. A health-care provider may prescribe this diet for your loved one if he does not eat enough protein or if additional protein is needed to rebuild tissue, such as skin.

Calorie-controlled diet. Your health-care provider may suggest a diet high in calories if your loved one needs to gain weight.

To lose weight, a low calorie diet should contain all the pro-

eating the food. In this case, your loved one must receive immediate emergency care. If your loved one has severe food allergies, the health-care provider may prescribe an epinephrine auto injector for your loved one.

teins, carbohydrates and fats your loved one needs. The health-care provider or dietitian may recommend a multivitamin containing mineral supplements.

Diabetic diet. If your loved one has type 1 or type 2 diabetes, the health-care provider may put your loved one on a special diet to help control blood glucose.

- Make sure your loved one eats about the same amount of carbohydrate foods each day.
- Provide meals and snacks at about the same times each day.
- Do not allow your loved one to skip meals or snacks.
- Make sure your loved one takes medications at the same times each day.
- Encourage your loved one to exercise at about the same time each day.

It is important to use a meal plan set up by a dietitian and pay special attention to the carbohydrates in the diet. Make sure your loved one eats a variety of the following foods:

- Low-fat milk and other low-fat dairy products
- Lean cuts of meat, chicken, fish
- Fresh fruits and vegetables
- Whole grain breads, cereals, rice, pasta and potatoes

Clear and Full Liquid Diets. Your health-care provider may recommend a clear liquid diet for only 1 or 2 days to give the digestive system a rest. A clear liquid diet includes liquids you can see through: broth, gelatin, carbonated beverages, tea, apple juice, grape juice and cranberry juice.

A full liquid diet includes orange juice, strained soups, ice cream, milk, diluted (thinned) cooked cereal, eggnog, supplements such as Carnation™ Instant Breakfast, Boost™ and Ensure.™

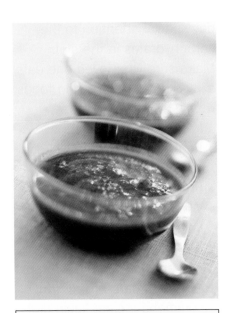

Pureed vegetables and meat are cooked and pureed in a blender or food processor.

similar to nectar or pudding. Always follow the directions on the container when using a thickening product.

Soft, Mechanical or Pureed Diet

A soft diet includes foods that are prepared soft or mashed, such as hot cereal, scrambled eggs, mashed potatoes or meatloaf.

A mechanical diet may include food, such as ground meat, that is finely chopped and diced with a knife or ground with a food processor.

Pureed food, such as pureed vegetables and meat, are cooked and pureed in a blender or food processor.

If you serve pureed food, separate each item on the plate so that it maintains a distinct identity from other pureed food you serve with it. Add seasoning to pureed food — using sauces, gravies and broths to give each item a good taste.

Thickened Liquids

If your loved one has problems swallowing liquids — such as fruit juice, milk, coffee, tea or soup — the health-care provider may suggest you thicken the beverages with a special thickener, such as Thick-It.™ Special thickeners make the drink's consistency

Low-Salt Diet

Salt often needs to be limited for people with high bood pressure or kidney or heart diseases. A low-salt diet includes foods that are low in sodium. Table salt may not be used, but a salt substitute may be used with the healthcare provider's approval.

Limit foods that are high in salt or sodium, such as ham, bacon, cheese, regular canned soups, potato chips, lunch meat, pickles and olives, frozen dinners and many packaged or canned foods.

Low-Fat Diet

A health-care provider may order a low-fat diet if your loved one has heart, gallbladder or liver disease. This diet calls for more protein and carbohydrates and restricted amounts of total fat.

Cut down on these 3 kinds of fat — saturated fat, trans fat and cholesterol. High amounts of saturated fat are found in animal products, such as fatty cuts of meat, chicken skin and in full-fat dairy products like butter, whole milk, cream and cheese and in tropical vegetable oils such as palm, palm kernel and coconut oil.

Trans fat is found in some of the same foods as saturated fat, such as vegetable shortening, some margarines (especially hard or stick margarine), crackers, cookies, baked goods, fried foods, salad dressings and other processed foods made with partially hydrogenated vegetable oils. Small amounts of trans fat also occur naturally in some animal products, such as milk products, beef and lamb.

Foods high in cholesterol include liver, other organ meats, egg yolks, shrimp and full-fat dairy products.

Renal Diet

If your loved one has kidney disease, then diet is important. The goal of a renal diet is to

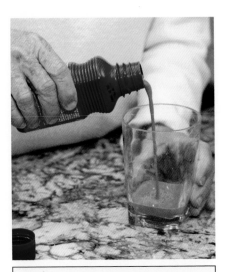

Some supplements are nutritionally complete meals.

Dietary Supplements

If your loved one has not been eating well or is losing weight because of an illness, the health-care provider may order a food supplement that is given with each meal or between meals. Some supplements are nutritionally complete meals.

Boost,™ Boost Plus,™ Ensure™ and Carnation™ Instant Breakfast are examples of food supplements. Your loved one may need a vitamin-mineral supplement to meet specific nutrition needs.

In addition to vitamins and minerals, dietary supplements include fiber, herbs and many other substances.

maintain nutrition, reduce the buildup of toxins and slow the progression of kidney disease. A dietitian specializing in renal nutrition can meet with you to plan meals for your loved one. Renal diets are often very complex and can restrict several nutrients. Visit the National Kidney Foundation Web site at www.kidney.org for additional information.

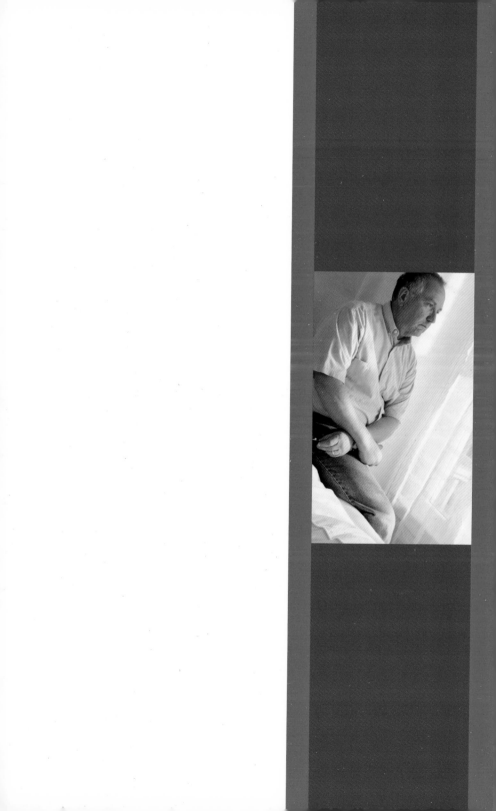

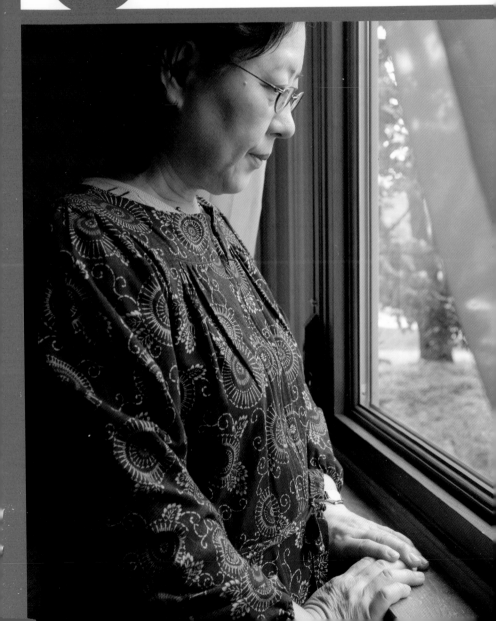

6

Caring for the Caregiver

"On my way home from the hospital after my heart attack all I could think about was my husband, Stuart," recalls Ellen, whose husband suffers from an aggressive, debilitating case of multiple sclerosis. "My doctor told me to take some time off to rest and recover. But how could I rest? The heart attack turned out to be a wake-up call for me. The MS Society helped us find a really good daily caregiver for Stuart who also helped with a good deal of the routine house-work. That ended up being a lifesaver for me."

tips

How to Cope with Stress

Here are some things you can do to relieve stress:

☐ Learn to let go. It's unrealistic to think you can do everything yourself. Make a list of tasks others can do, such as cleaning the house, grocery shopping, preparing meals or running errands.

☐ Ask for help. Don't wait for others to offer; they may not know what you need. Talk with your family on a regular basis about the many responsibilities involved in your loved one's care and ask each person to commit to help.

Stress

Caring for a loved one can be rewarding but it's also time-consuming. For most caregivers, there are never enough hours in the day.

The physical and emotional strain of family illness and your caregiving responsibilities can cause stress, depression, anxiety and even physical illness.

Learn the Symptoms

Learn to recognize stress early and take your needs seriously, so you can make changes to help yourself. Here are some signs:

Physical Symptoms
- Sleep disturbances
- Back, shoulder or neck pain
- Tension or migraine headaches
- Stomach and/or bowel ailments
- Weight gain or loss, eating disorders
- Hair loss
- Muscle tension

- Fatigue
- High blood pressure
- Irregular heartbeat, palpitations
- Asthma or shortness of breath
- Chest pain
- Sweaty palms or hands
- Cold hands or feet
- Skin problems (hives, eczema, psoriasis, itching)
- Immune system suppression: more colds, flu, infections

Emotional Symptoms

- Nervousness, anxiety
- Depression, moodiness
- Irritability, frustration
- Memory problems
- Lack of concentration
- Trouble thinking clearly
- Feeling out of control
- Substance abuse
- Phobias
- Overreactions

Relational Symptoms

- Increased arguments
- Isolation from social activities
- Conflict with co-workers or employers

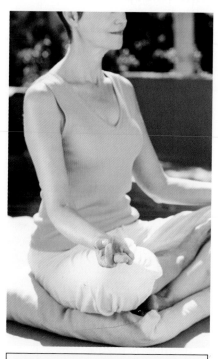

Mild exercise and yoga are great stress relievers.

- Frequent job changes
- Road rage
- Domestic or workplace violence
- Overreactions

While these symptoms are common in caregivers, they

tips

How to Cope
with Stress

- [ ] Get help from community groups, such as respite care services or faith-based organizations. Respite services may be offered through local hospitals, long-term care facilities or assisted-living facilities.
- [ ] Express your feelings. Emotions are a normal part of being human. Share your feelings with other family members. If your feelings make you uncomfortable, talk with a professional, such as a health-care provider, psychologist or clergy.

are not healthy. These are warning signs that you need help. Some of these symptoms could also be signs of depression.

Employee Assistance Programs

In addition to caregiving responsibilities, most caregivers work outside of the home. Many corporations offer benefits for employees who care for a family member. These benefits may include employee assistance programs, flextime or personal leaves of absence. The Family Medical Leave Act ensures that your employer must give you your job back if you have to take some time off to care for a family member. Talk with your human resources representative about this and other programs your company may offer.

Respite Care

Respite services can provide a substantial amount of help for your loved one. These services range from volunteer services, adult daycare, a short-term stay in a nursing home or assisted-living facility for your loved one, a home health aide, a private-duty nurse or adult foster care.

Respite care can also be provided by a friend or family member who can stay with your loved one to give you a short break to attend to other things, go to a health-care provider's appointment, go shopping, take a nap, see a movie, take a vacation or simply visit with friends or family. You might consider scheduling some respite care services on

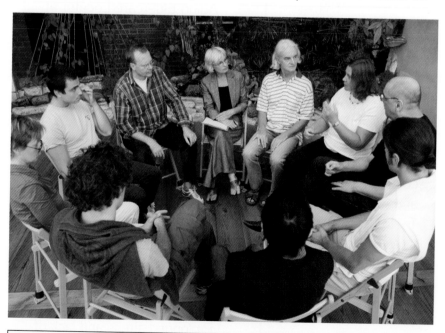

Joining a caregivers' support group will help you understand what you are going through and will help you feel less isolated.

tips

How to Cope with Stress

- ☐ Develop a care calendar showing who will assist with your loved one's care and when. This will help you plan ahead.
- ☐ Join a caregivers' support group. Talking with others who understand what you are going through will help you feel less isolated. This will also provide a helpful network where you can share ideas and information about community resources and equipment.
- ☐ Try to get 7 to 8 hours of sleep every night. When you can't, try to take a nap during the day.

an ongoing basis for your loved one to give yourself a much-needed regular break.

The federal Administration on Aging often works through state and area agencies on aging, adult daycare centers and other organizations to help provide respite services. Call your local Area Agency on Aging Eldercare Locator at 800-677-1116.

Some faith-based organizations offer programs and services for caregivers, in which volunteers can sit with your loved one while you do other things.

Depression

When your loved one is ill and recovery is uncertain, it's normal to be worried, sad and afraid. Your loved one may behave in ways that are difficult to handle. Providing care may mean that you aren't getting enough sleep. Prolonged stress and lack of sleep can lead to depression. Here are some of the symptoms:

- Persistent sad, anxious or "empty" mood
- Feelings of hopelessness, pessimism
- Feelings of guilt, worthlessness, helplessness
- Loss of interest or pleasure in hobbies and activities that were once enjoyed, including sex
- Decreased energy, fatigue, being "slowed down"
- Difficulty concentrating, remembering, making decisions
- Insomnia, early-morning awakening or oversleeping
- Appetite and/or weight loss or overeating and weight gain
- Thoughts of death or suicide; suicide attempts
- Restlessness, irritability
- Persistent physical symptoms that do not respond to treatment, such as headaches, digestive disorders and chronic pain

Not everyone who is depressed experiences every symptom. If you think you have depression, or are feeling down, see your health-care provider and/or a mental health professional, such as a psychologist or psychiatrist. Let him or her know that you care for a loved one and how you have been feeling.

Your health insurance and Medicare should cover some mental health care. Check with your health insurance provider for a list of mental health professionals who accept your insurance.

Dealing with Depression

The National Institute of Mental Health offers these suggestions for dealing with depression:

- Set realistic goals and don't try to take on more responsibility than you can handle.
- Break large tasks into small ones, set priorities and do what you can as you can.

tips

How to Cope with Stress

☐ Try to get regular exercise for at least 30 minutes two to three times a week. Mild exercise is a great stress reliever and it helps regulate sleep.

☐ Find a reason to laugh often. Watch a funny movie, read a funny story or see a comedy act. Like exercise, laughter releases chemicals in your body that help relieve stress.

☐ Set aside time for yourself each day. Read a book, get a massage, see a friend or go to the gym.

☐ Use the employee assistance program at your workplace (see page 90).

- Try to be with other people and to confide in someone.
- Participate in activities that may make you feel better, such as mild exercise, going to a movie or ballgame, or attending a religious, social or community event.
- Expect your mood to improve gradually, not immediately. People rarely "snap out of" depression. But they can feel a little better each day.
- It is best to postpone important decisions until the depression has lifted. Before deciding to make a significant transition — change jobs, get married or divorced — discuss it with others who know you well and have a more objective view of your situation.
- Let your family and friends help you.

Accept Your Feelings

Feelings of anger, frustration, sadness and guilt are normal when caring for a loved one with an illness. If you are caring for a parent, you both may have to define your roles and adjust to having closer contact or living in the same house once again. You may feel resentful or irritated by your loved one's behavior. Caregivers often feel frustrated because even though they provide the best care they can, their loved one may not get better. Frustration can lead to anger and anger to guilt.

- Talk with friends, family, a counselor, clergy or a health professional about your feelings.
- Write about your feelings in a journal. Writing can be therapeutic and can help you release negative feelings.

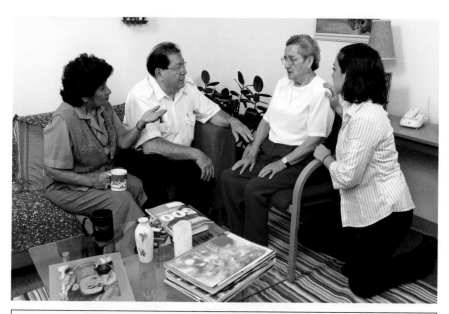

Talk with friends, family, a counselor, clergy or a health professional about your feelings.

- If you feel sad, give yourself permission to cry.
- When angry, leave the room to cool off for a few minutes, if possible. Try punching a pillow — this is a healthy release that won't hurt anyone.
- Do not expect perfection from yourself or others.

- Handle each situation as well as you can and learn from your mistakes.
- Do not dwell on things that have gone wrong.

End of Life Issues

When your loved one reaches the end of life, caring for him or

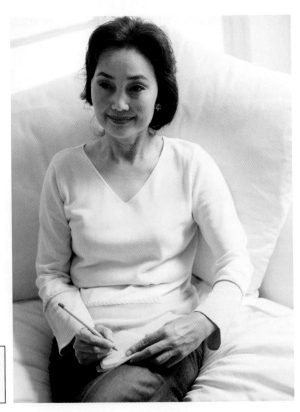

Write about your feelings in a journal.

her can become more difficult, emotionally and physically. In the final days, body functions will begin to fail and he or she may have pain or may be unconscious. During this time you will rely heavily on the help and support of family, friends and community organizations, such as a hospice. Call on friends and family to give you the support you need during this emotional time.

Hospice Care

When health-care professionals can do no more for a loved one's terminal illness, you may find that hospice care can help you when your loved one reaches the final days of her life. Hospice care provides support for you and your family while making sure that your loved one is comfortable and without pain. Hospice care can take place at home or in a special unit in the hospital. For additional information on hospice care, contact the National Hospice and Palliative Care Organization at 800-658-8898 or visit www.nhpco.org.

Dealing with Loss

Dr. Elizabeth Kubler-Ross identified 5 stages of emotions a dying person – and his loved ones – may experience. Not everyone goes through all 5 stages, and every person goes through each stage at his or her own pace. You may experience these stages yourself, or see them in your family, close friends and the person in your care.

Denial. People often insist their loved one is not terminally ill. They cannot accept something as terrible as having a terminal illness or having someone they love die. A period of denial is a time of emotional shock that causes people to delay dealing with it until they are emotionally ready.

Anger. You, your loved one and your family members may express anger as a symptom of underlying emotions such as fear, resentment and frustration. Anger is often directed towards people with whom we are closest and it can be sparked by something that seems trivial. Or, anger may be directed at God in such statements as: "What did I do to deserve this?"

It is important to not take angry remarks personally, but rather try to identify the underlying emotion to better understand what is really being expressed.

Bargaining. A person may try to bargain for more time by making a deal, usually with God. For example, a person may say something like: "Just let me make it to my daughter's wedding; I won't ask for anything else."

Depression. Depression during the dying process can take two forms:
1. Grief over past losses, disappointments and unfulfilled dreams
2. Preparation for losses to come..

Listen to each other and accept expressions of sorrow during this time.

As a caregiver, you may be the only person others talk to about grief and dying. Do not try to cheer the depressed person, offer distraction from grief or try to persuade him to feel grateful about what went right in his life. Seek out someone who can listen to you as well.

Sometimes a family member may withdraw or become detached, as if he has lost interest in everything other than his own comfort. This is a more common reaction among men, who may feel they do not have permission to cry or grieve.

Acceptance. This period of calm happens when the person reaches an emotional stage of peaceful resignation and lets go of the need to fight the inevitable movement from health to sickness or from life to death.

People often move back and forth between stages, instead of progressing straight through them. Your role as a caregiver is not to try to help people move through these stages towards acceptance, but to be aware of your own normal feelings and those of others. Be kind. Accept these feelings and try to understand.

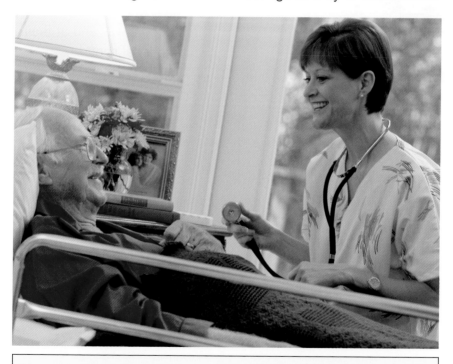

You may find that hospice can help your loved one when he reaches the final days of his life.

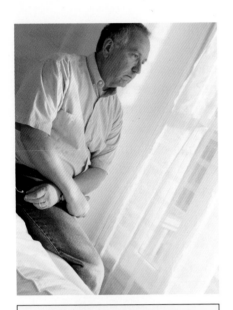

Hear what others need to express at that moment without making argumentative or judgmental remarks.

Get help for yourself. Caregivers need to understand their own feelings of loss and avoid overreacting to other people's feelings. Everyone must deal with grief in their own personal way and at their own emotional speed.

Acceptance is a period of calm when a person reaches peaceful resignation.

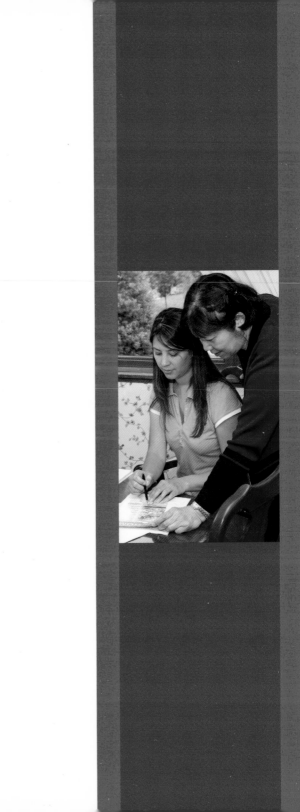

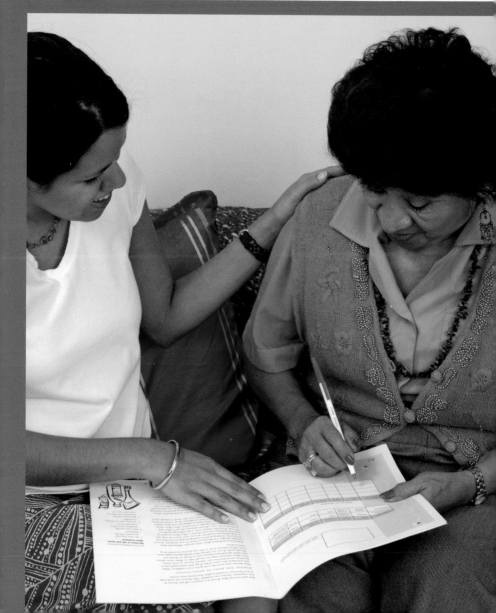

Legal and Financial Issues

"**W**hen Mom was diagnosed with Parkinson's disease, a social worker at the hospital recommended that I have her sign the legal documents I would need to take care of her affairs when she could no longer do this for herself," recalls Maria. "Otherwise, I eventually might be forced to go to court — a painful and expensive legal process I wanted to avoid."

Gather Important Documents

Caring for your loved one may involve making important legal decisions, especially if he becomes dependent. Help him gather and organize important documents such as a will, insurance papers, business records, income tax records, health-care history and other business or financial records.

Keep a list of these documents and know where they can be found. All documents should be secured at an accessible location that is protected from damage or theft.

You may also want to ask your loved one if he would like to make plans now for a time in the future when he may not be capable of making his own decisions. The topic can bring up sensitive issues for some people so approach the subject delicately.

Advance Directives

Advance directives enable your loved one to document his wishes about such things as medical care and who should handle his affairs in advance, in case he becomes unable to make those decisions. These documents include:

- **A living will** that specifies the medical treatment your loved one wishes to receive when he is facing death. This can include a variety of instructions.
- **A durable medical power of attorney** enables your loved one to appoint a person to make health-care decisions on his behalf if he becomes unable to do so. These decisions may be about the types of medical treatment he wants, or doesn't want, to receive and end-of-life care.
- **A Do Not Resuscitate (DNR)** order instructs emergency responders to not use cardiopulmonary resuscitation (CPR) if breathing or heartbeat stops. It must be

signed by your doctor and kept with your loved one.

- **A durable power of attorney for finances** appoints someone to make financial decisions when a person is unable to do so.

A *durable* power of attorney remains effective even if your loved one becomes incapacitated or mentally incompetent.

Advance directives help ensure your loved one's care will be consistent with *his* wishes if he becomes too sick to make those decisions or is not of sound mind at that time.

Without a living will and a

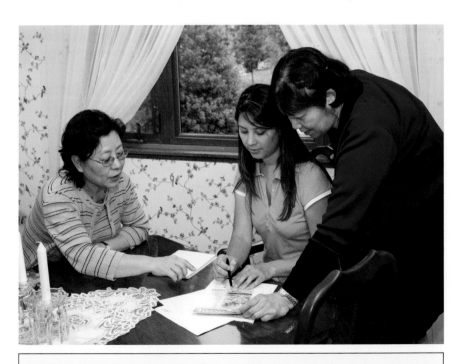

It's important that your loved one's advance directives be shared with close family members and health-care professionals.

durable medical power of attorney, family members and health-care providers will have to guess about a person's preferences if he is unable to communicate them.

Getting Help with Advance Directives

If your loved one wants to create a living will or to give you or someone else medical or financial power of attorney, you or your loved one should talk with your loved one's doctor, a representative at your local Area Agency on Aging or an attorney to get helpful forms and advice. They can help make sure your loved one's wishes are understandable and consistent with your state laws.

In some states, advanced directives need only be signed, dated, copied and distributed to the health-care provider and family members.

It is important that your loved one's advance directives be shared with close family members and health-care professionals. Keep them in an accessible place so you can show them to health-care professionals if your loved one becomes unable to speak for himself.

Advance directives may be revised at any time. In some states, your loved one only needs to sign and date the new ones and they will be effective.

Last Will and Testament

A will is a legal document that specifies how a person's property and personal assets are to be divided after death. It should be updated periodically to reflect changes in family, the estate or valuable items.

When a person dies without a will, the family often has to pay higher estate taxes and legal fees. Moreover, property and assets are transferred according to state laws that may not be consistent with the wishes of the person.

When creating a will, consider helping others by signing up with an organ donation program.

Facts About Funerals

Unless your loved one has made funeral arrangements in advance, when he dies you and the rest of his family will be faced with many questions.

Many people feel uncomfortable comparing prices and negotiating over the funeral costs after having just lost a loved one. But funerals are expensive and you may choose to compare prices. Ask the funeral providers for a price list and choose the specific services you want. You do not have to buy a package

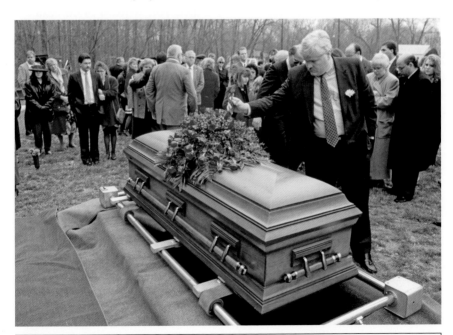

Making final arrangements in advance can spare family members from having to make difficult decisions at an emotional time.

that includes items or services you do not want.

If your loved one intends to be buried in another state, find out in advance if there are state regulations about transporting a deceased person across state lines.

Recognize your rights. Laws regarding funerals and burials vary from state to state. It's wise to know which products or services the law requires and which ones are optional.

For more information about planning or preplanning a funeral, visit the Web site of the National Funeral Directors Association at www.nfda.org.

Tips to Remember When Planning a Funeral

The Federal Trade Commission (FTC) offers the following tips when planning a funeral:

- Ask for a price list. The law requires funeral homes to give you written price lists for products and services.
- Avoid emotional overspending. Resist pressure to buy products and services you don't really want or need.

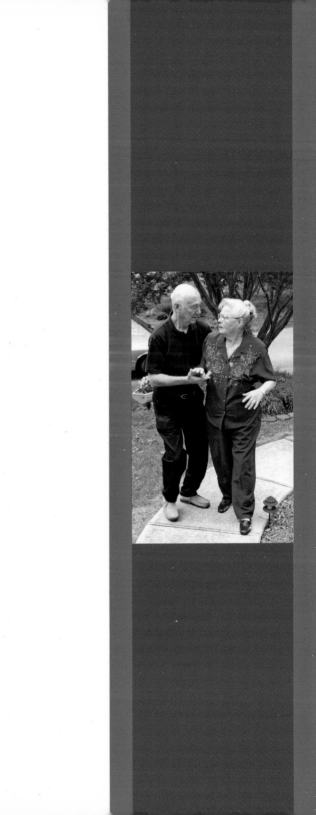

8

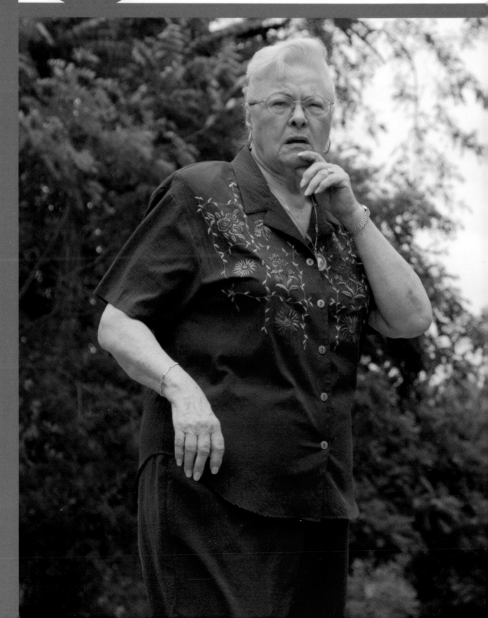

Dementia

"One of the frustrating things I often dealt with when taking care of mom was her frequent insistence that she wanted to talk to 'John' about something," recalls Beverly. "Sadly, John, her husband — my father — had been dead for nearly a decade. But no matter how many times I reminded Mom about that, she continued to insist — often several times a day — that she had to talk to him. Eventually, I realized that it was probably because she missed him. So instead of trying to correct her, I suggested we look at a photo album that had pictures of Dad. That often eased her anxiety and allowed us to enjoy some fond memories of Dad together."

Dealing with Difficult Behaviors

As a caregiver, you may find yourself having to deal with difficult behavior. This is especially true if your loved one suffers from dementia which affects not only memory but also thinking, judgment and impulse control. Your loved one with dementia has the same basic needs as everyone else, but cognitive decline impairs her ability to meet those needs for herself, or even express her needs to others.

Many caregivers find it helpful to join support groups where common experiences, feelings, concerns and ideas for dealing with difficulties are shared openly. It will be easier — and less stressful — for you to deal with your loved one's difficult behavior if you know what to expect and how to respond effectively. When your loved one behaves in a dysfunctional way, think of the behavior as a form of communication. Your loved one is trying to tell you, in the only way she can, that something is wrong. Watch her closely and think about the behavior. You may not always be able to help, but you may find out what she is trying to tell you so you can provide appropriate care.

Some common behavior patterns for people with dementia are:
- Pacing and wandering
- Rummaging and hoarding
- Overreacting to situations (often called a *catastrophic reaction*)
- Increased restlessness and confusion as evening approaches (often called *sundowning*)

Pacing and Wandering
Your loved one may walk aimlessly in an area and then walk or wander away. This behavior — which can be unsafe — often is a response to being over-stimulated by too much talking

or noise; feeling uncomfortable, anxious or disoriented;
looking for someone or something; or feeling unhappy about
what is happening.

Try these suggestions:

- Reassure your loved one.
  Listen for a clue about what
  she is trying to communicate.
  Gently ask, "May I walk with
  you?" and guide your loved
  one back to where she
  should be.
- A distraction may help.
  Offer a snack, take her for a
  walk or do something she
  likes to do.
- Take your loved one to the
  bathroom. She may have a
  full bladder and not realize it.
- Try to help remove your
  loved one's shoes. Removing
  shoes may prompt an old
  memory that taking off
  shoes means a person
  should sit or lie down.
- Observe your loved one for
  signs of anxiety (i.e., restlessness, fidgeting). Give her a

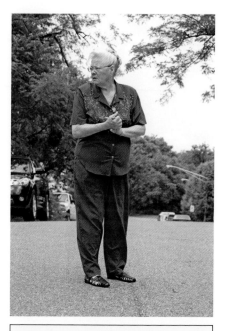

Wandering can be a response
to feeling uncomfortable,
anxious or disoriented.

ball or another smooth object
to manipulate in her hands.
Report these symptoms to
your loved one's health-care
provider at the next visit.

- Talk to your loved one and
  listen to what she says.
- Take these 3 steps to
  prevent your confused loved

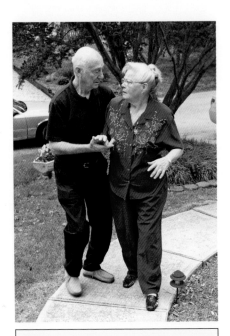

When a loved one wanders, guide her back to where she should be.

doors to alert you if your loved one tries to leave.

- Have her wear a metal bracelet imprinted with her name, address, phone number and the words "Memory Impaired." Place a card with this information in her pocket and keep a recent photograph or videotape of your loved one to show searchers if she gets lost.

- Register your loved one with the Alzheimer's Association Safe Return program. Visit www.alz.org or call 888-572-8566.

- Register your loved one with the local police department and notify them right away if she becomes lost. Leave a phone number where you can be reached if she is found.

one from leaving the house unsupervised.

1. Make sure she does not have access to the car.

2. Hang mirrors on all house exit doors to help camouflage them.

3. Consider installing an alarm on all house exit

Rummaging and Hoarding

Rummaging and hoarding can be signs that your loved one feels generally lost and confused, or not able to find something she wants. Here are some suggestions to help you respond:

- Do not scold your loved one for her actions because she may become fearful of you.
- Try distracting her with another activity or a snack.
- Show your loved one where her personal belongings are.
- Take her to the bathroom. (She may have been searching for it.)
- Learn her hiding places so you can find lost items.
- Use your sense of fun and humor to help your loved one enjoy her environment, but be careful not to laugh at her behavior.
- Label her personal items and provide specific places for them. Put valuables away.
- Keep a spare set of keys in a safe place.
- Provide a rummaging drawer of safe items such as books, an old wallet, small toys or coins through which she can freely look.

Catastrophic Reactions

When your loved one is overwhelmed by a situation, she may overreact because the ability to control impulses is lost. This is called a *catastrophic reaction*. Some people may even strike out at others. When responding to a catastrophic reaction, try these suggestions:

- Identify yourself as you approach her.
- Do not take the attack personally.
- Avoid arguing.
- Keep routines as structured, predictable and orderly as possible.
- Stay calm, even if you are unable to control your loved one's actions.
- Prevent her from becoming injured or injuring anyone else, but do not restrain her.
- Acknowledge her anger by saying something like, "You seem upset. What is upsetting you?" Wait for a verbal

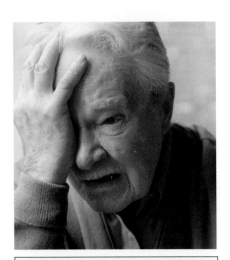

Signs of sundowning can include anxiety, crying or pushing others away.

does not respond to you, try giving her a warm bath or backrub to calm her.

Sundowning

As late afternoon or evening approaches, many people become tired and less able to handle stress. You may notice your loved one becomes more restless, confused, demanding, upset, suspicious or disoriented. This behavior, called *sundowning*, is common in people with dementia.

Sundowning is a symptom of her condition over which she has no control.

Towards evening, the increasing darkness may cause her to feel confused or afraid. Signs of sundowning can include restlessness, anxiety, worried expressions, reluctance to enter her room, reluctance to enter brightly lit areas, crying, wringing hands, pushing others away, gritting teeth or removing clothing.

or nonverbal response after each question.

- Reassure your loved one that you aren't going to hurt her, and won't allow her to hurt anyone.
- Let her know the limits by saying something such as, "It's not okay to hit someone. It hurts."
- Distract her with her favorite activity. If your loved one still

These signs may be your loved one's way of telling you that she needs something. She may need to use the bathroom, or she may be uncomfortable or in pain. It might also mean that she wants family and other human contact for comfort or to feel that she has control over something.

Other common behaviors may include saying things that don't make sense, seeing or hearing things that aren't real, believing things that aren't true, being depressed or angry and being suspicious of other people.

When responding to signs of sundowning, try this:

- First, determine whether your loved one has any physical needs, such as going to the bathroom or eating.
- Look for other clues that reveal her emotional needs. Does she look worried? She may be afraid of the dark or of unfamiliar sounds, or of being left alone. Accept your loved one's feelings.
- Provide enough light for your loved one to see her surroundings, but avoid glaring, bright lights that cast harsh shadows.
- Talk softly to your loved one and try to soothe her by rubbing her arm or back. Having something to cuddle and listening to soothing music may comfort her.
- Going for an early evening walk may help your loved one feel calmer.
- Try using distraction; a temporary change of subject or scene often solves the problem.

Comforting a Loved One with Dementia

Understanding how to comfort your loved one will help both of you feel less stressed and may help you feel less overwhelmed by unwanted behavior. It will also help you provide safe and compassionate care as

tips

Communicating

- [ ] Stand directly in front of your loved one and maintain eye contact.
- [ ] Touching her arm or shoulder gently may help her stay focused.
- [ ] Speak softly, slowly and clearly, using simple words and sentences. If your loved one doesn't understand, patiently repeat the words.
- [ ] Use direct statements when you want your loved one to do something. For example, "It's time to eat breakfast now."

you prepare for the road ahead.

Your loved one still needs joy and pleasure in life. Simple pleasures such as a warm comfortable bed, a gentle massage, soft music, sweet smells and bright colors can add to the quality of your loved one's life.

Focus on Surroundings

Create surroundings that are restful and stress-free. Learn how to communicate with her so that she understands you, and recognize the ways she tries to communicate with you.

Keep your loved one's surroundings and activities orderly and safe.

Focus on Kindness

Treat your loved one gently, sensitively and with respect. You can provide better care if she knows you care about her and are trying to understand and help her.

If your loved one has difficulty

with things she once knew how to do, show her how to do them again. Praise your loved one's actions as often as possible.

Focus on Quiet
When your loved one is agitated or confused, talk softly and eliminate as much noise as possible.

Focus on Calmness
If your loved one is agitated or wandering, help her relax and satisfy her need for motion by encouraging her to sit in a comfortable rocking chair.

Giving her something soft to hug, such as a stuffed animal, may help calm her. Try playing slow-tempo, classical music softly in the background.

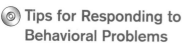 **Tips for Responding to Behavioral Problems**

- When your loved one behaves in a way that seems inappropriate, don't confront or accuse her. Her understanding of the world is

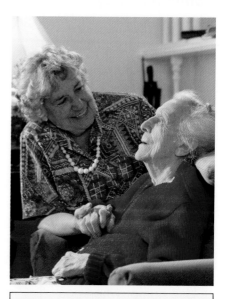

When speaking to your loved one, maintain eye contact.

different than it once was.
- Follow a simple, set routine; frequent changes can be confusing.
- Avoid situations that could make your loved one angry or frustrated.
- Demonstrate activities in small steps. She may only be able to pay attention for a short time.

tips

◉ Communicating

- [ ] Allow extra time for your loved one to understand and answer. Don't expect a quick response to a question or statement. If you don't get an answer, then ask the question again using the exact words, or come back 5 or 10 minutes later and ask again.
- [ ] Use humor when possible and appropriate.
- [ ] Because your loved one with dementia is often more comfortable in her own reality, don't argue or confront her. If she believes that it's 1956 and she is 19 years old, don't correct her unless she is unhappy or anxious. Respond to her emotions, not to the facts.

◉ Doing Activities

It is worth the effort to find easy and interesting activities your loved one can do. Choose simple activities, such as sorting yarn by color or folding socks. Avoid teaching a new skill if it frustrates your loved one.

Help your loved one begin an activity by showing her what to do. If your loved one gets frustrated with an activity, gently help or distract her with something else.

Do different activities throughout the day. For example, after breakfast, talk about pleasant events in the newspaper. After lunch, work in the garden or go for a walk. In the evening, watch a show on television or look through a magazine.

Exercise

It is very beneficial to exercise 30 minutes per day doing such activities as walking, dancing, or gardening. Studies have shown that even a modest amount of exercise reduces stress, improves well-being and even increases life expectancy.

Exercise is good for both you and your loved one, so try to make it a part of your daily routine. You may prefer to spread out your exercise throughout the day — mixing active chores, like walking out to the mailbox and emptying the trash, with other things you may enjoy, like a walk in the park or easy weight-training. If mobility is a problem for your loved one, try doing chair exercises.

Wear comfortable clothes and good walking shoes. Warm up for 5 minutes at the begin-

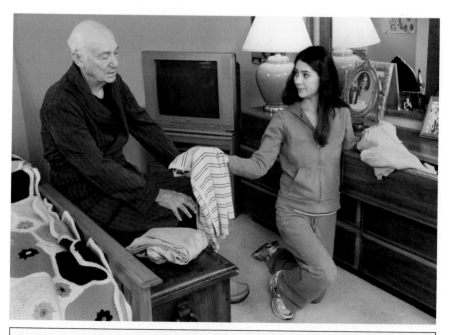

Choose simple activities, such as sorting yarn by color or folding laundry.

ning of any activity. Walking slowly and stretching are good warm-up activities. After first checking with your doctor, start a mild exercise program slowly and don't expect your loved one to do too much all at once. Also, stop if your loved one shows any signs of discomfort or stress.

Sleeping

Many older people have trouble sleeping. If your loved one does not want to go to sleep or does not stay in bed, try to keep bedtime about the same time each evening and create a quiet, calm environment. Dim the lights and play soothing music. Offer only non-caffeinated beverages in the afternoon and evening.

You may find that a daily mild exercise routine makes your loved one physically tired and helps her sleep better.

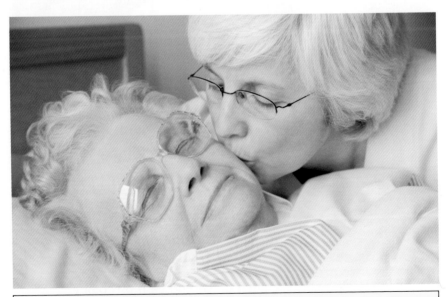

Create a quiet, calm environment at bedtime for your loved one.

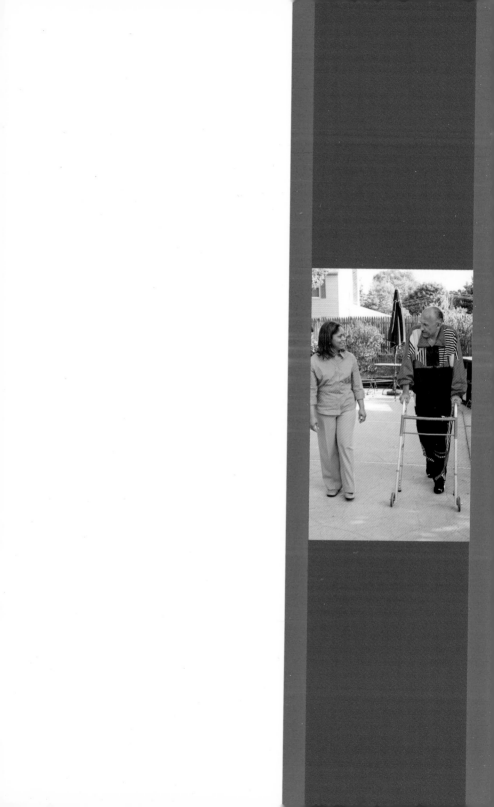

9

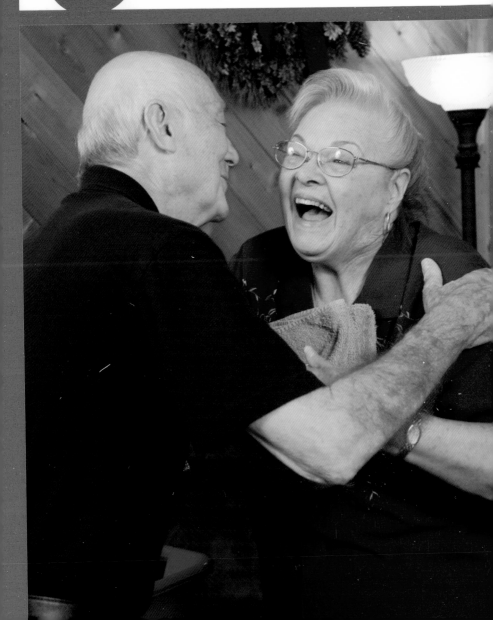

Caregiving Resources

"Having respite care for my wife a few days a week gives me a much needed break," says Joe. "I feel refreshed and better able to enjoy my time with Suzanne."

Local and National Organizations

Local Organizations
The Eldercare Locator is the best place to find phone numbers and websites of *local* community services that can help you and your loved one.

Eldercare Locator
800-677-1116
9:00 a.m. to 8:00 p.m., ET; M-F
www.eldercare.gov.

National Organizations

AARP
888-687-2277;
7:00 a.m. to 12:00 p.m., ET; M-F
www.aarp.org

Administration on Aging
202-619-0724
www.aoa.gov
(multiple languages)

Alzheimer's Association
800-272-3900
(24-hour caregiver help line)
www.alz.org

American Diabetes Association
800-342-2383;
8:30 a.m. to 8 p.m., ET; M-F
www.diabetes.org

American Red Cross
Call your local chapter.
www.redcross.org

Benefits CheckUP
www.benefitscheckup.org

Caregivers Marketplace
800-888-0889
or 866-327-8340
www.caregiversmarketplace.com

Centers for Disease Control and Prevention (CDC)
800-311-3435
www.cdc.gov

Family Caregiver Alliance
800-445-8106
www.caregiver.org

Lifeline®
800-959-6989
www.lifelinesys.com

**Meals on Wheels
Association of America**
Call Eldercare Locator:
800-677-1116
www.mowaa.org

Medicare
800-MEDICARE,
800 633-2273
(24 hour hotline)
www.medicare.gov

**National Alliance
for Caregiving**
E-mail: info@caregiving.org
www.caregiving.org

National Cancer Institute
800-4-CANCER
or 800-422-6237
9:00 a.m. to 4:30 p.m., ET; M-F
www.cancer.gov

**National Family
Caregivers Association**
800-896-3650
9 a.m. to 5 p.m., ET; M-F
www.thefamilycaregiver.org

**National Hospice and
Palliative Care Organization**
800-658-8898 (helpline)
www.nhpco.org

National Institute on Aging
800-222-2225
8:30 a.m. to 5:00 p.m., ET; M-F
www.nia.nih.gov

**National Respite
Locator Service**
919-490-5577
(select voice mail option
for ARCH)
www.respitelocator.org

**Rosalynn Carter
Institute for Caregiving**
229-928-1234
www.RosalynnCarter.org

Strength for Caring
866-466-3458
www.strengthforcaring.com

Vital Signs Record

This chart may be helpful if your loved one's health-care provider suggests keeping a record of his vital signs.

Date	Time	Temp.	Pulse	Respiration	Blood Pressure

Daily Medication Log

Use the checklist below to keep track of each dose of medicine your loved one takes. You may also find daily or weekly medicine containers (available at most drug stores) help you and your loved one remember to take each dose.

Date	Medication Name and Dosage	Morn.	Noon	Eve.	Bed Time

Medication List

Keep a medications list for your loved one and take it with you when you go to the health care provider.

Date	Medication Name and Number	Dosage	When Taken	Medical Condition Treated	Prescribing Physician	When Started	Special Instructions or Precautions	Refills

American Red Cross Emergency Contact Card

Directions:

1. Make a photocopy of this card for each family member.

2. Cut out the card along the dotted lines.

3. Write contact information of those who should be called in the event of an emergency, include home, work and cellular phone numbers.

4. After discussing with other family members, also write who will be contacted and where your family will gather in the event of a regional disaster. (For more information on how to create a family disaster plan and assemble an emergency supplies kit, as well as other valuable preparedness information, visit www.redcross.org.)

5. On the back of the card, list current medical conditions and medications — both prescription and over-the-counter.

6. Fold the card so it fits in your pocket, wallet or purse.

7. Carry this card with you at all times so you — or emergency medical responders — will have quick access to vital information if it is needed.

Visit www.redcross.org for more information

Other:

Other:

Poison Control Center: 1-800-222-1222

Family Doctor:

Ambulance: Call 9-1-1 or

Fire Dept.: Call 9-1-1 or

Police: Call 9-1-1 or

Important Phone Numbers

Emergency Contact Card

American Red Cross

Name:

Home Address:

Phone Number:

Family Members Contact Information

Doctor(s):

Out-of-town contact:

Family meeting place outside the neighborhood:

FOLD

FOLD

FOLD

Medical Conditions

_____
_____
_____
_____
_____
_____
_____
_____

FOLD —

_____
_____
_____
_____
_____
_____
_____
_____
_____

FOLD —

Medications

_____ ☐ Rx ☐ OTC
_____ ☐ Rx ☐ OTC
_____ ☐ Rx ☐ OTC
_____ ☐ Rx ☐ OTC
_____ ☐ Rx ☐ OTC

FOLD —

_____ ☐ Rx ☐ OTC
_____ ☐ Rx ☐ OTC
_____ ☐ Rx ☐ OTC
_____ ☐ Rx ☐ OTC
_____ ☐ Rx ☐ OTC

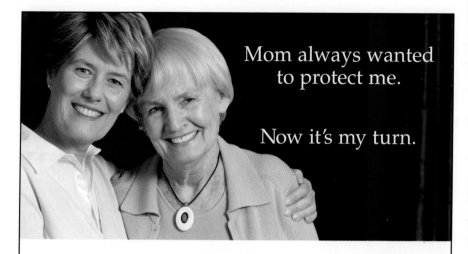

Mom always wanted to protect me.

Now it's my turn.

We've all heard the stories.

Somebody's mother or grandmother had a fall. And because they lived by themselves, they ended up lying there, alone and helpless.

The first thought is always, "what if that were Mom?" After all those years of your parents worrying about you, now your find yourself worrying about them.

But there is a way to help your loved ones keep their independence, while you maintain a little peace of mind. It's called Lifeline®.

Make living alone safer, 24 hours a day.

Lifeline is a medical alert designed to reduce the risk of living alone. In the event of a fall or emergency, help is available at the push of a button.

Personal Help Button

The Lifeline Personal Help Button connects your loved one to a trained Personal Response Associate who can send help quickly – 24 hours a day, 7 days a week.

American Red Cross offers the Lifeline service to support its mission of helping families prevent, prepare for and respond to emergencies.

Don't wait for a fall or medical emergency. Contact the American Red Cross to get Lifeline for someone you care about and ease your worried mind.

For more information,

call 1-800-959-6989
and refer to <u>code 44</u>

or visit www.redcross.org

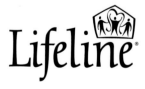

Lifeline®

For us, CPR is a family thing.

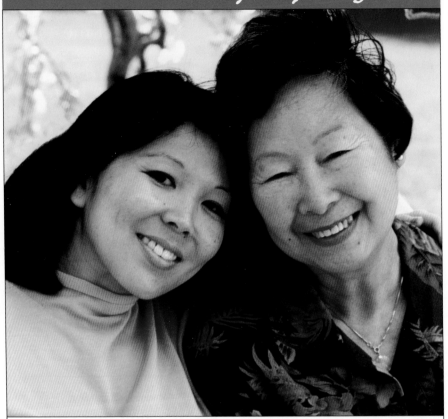

Shortly after Mom moved in with us, she collapsed from a heart attack. But thanks to my Red Cross training, I knew just what to do. Now Mom is back on her feet again enjoying life.

Nothing brings peace of mind like being prepared.

CPR saves lives. Protect your loved ones with the best in first aid and CPR training from the American Red Cross.

Learn how to save a life—contact your local American Red Cross chapter or visit www.redcross.org today!

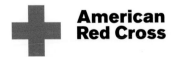

American Red Cross